Antimicrobial therapy in swine
A practical approach

Copyright © 2013 Grupo Asís Biomedia, SL
Plaza Antonio Beltrán Martínez nº 1, planta 8 - letra I
(Centro empresarial El Trovador)
50002 Zaragoza - Spain

First edition: July 2013
Second edition: April 2016

Illustrators:
Jacob Gragera Artal

ISBN: 978-84-941014-9-6
DL: Z 1090-2013

Design, layout and printing:
Servet editorial - Grupo Asís Biomedia, SL
www.grupoasis.com
info@grupoasis.com

Servet is the publishing house of Grupo Asís

Warning:

Veterinary science is constantly evolving, as are pharmacology and the other sciences. Inevitably, it is therefore the responsibility of the veterinary surgeon to determine and verify the dosage, the method of administration, the duration of treatment and any possible contraindications to the treatments given to each individual patient, based on his or her professional experience. Neither the publisher nor the author can be held liable for any damage or harm caused to people, animals or properties resulting from the correct or incorrect application of the information contained in this book.

Antimicrobial therapy in swine

A PRACTICAL APPROACH

Lorenzo Fraile

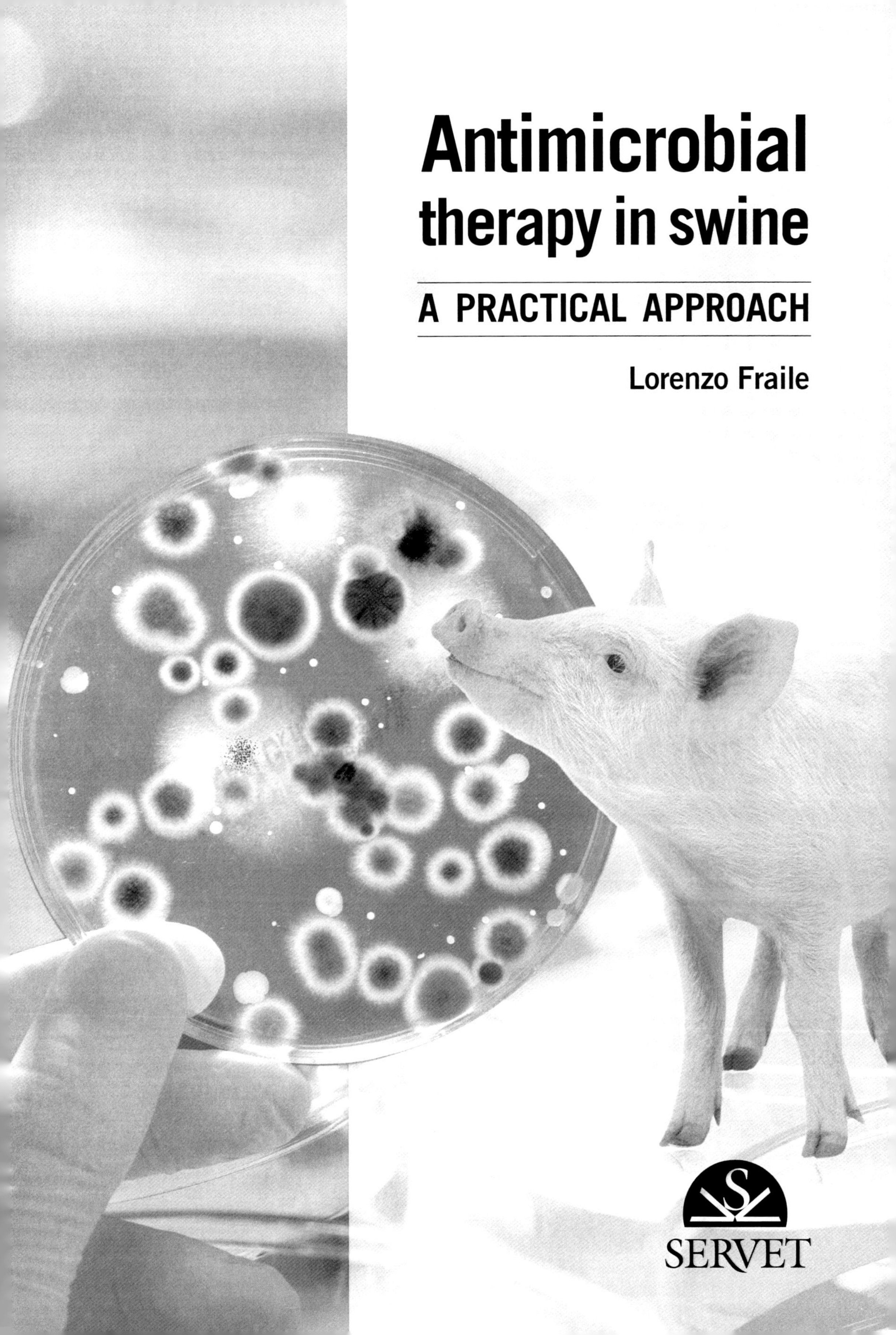

SERVET

This book is dedicated to
my family—Pily, Pablo and Teresa—,
whose sacrifice and love have made
this book possible.

Acknowledgments

I would like to express my gratitude to:

The members of the Department of Pharmacology of the University of Zaragoza, who instilled in me a love for pharmacology and teaching.

Don Santiago Bernaus Español and Don Santiago Bernaus i Gaset, who gave me the opportunity to work for their company (Picber, S.A.) and for their confidence in my work for many years.

Dr Joaquim Segalés, who provided many photographs for this book.

Dr John Mackinnon, who actively participated in the chapter on the prudent use of antimicrobials.

The members of the Servet Editorial team, for their help and for making my life a bit easier on so many occasions.

Author

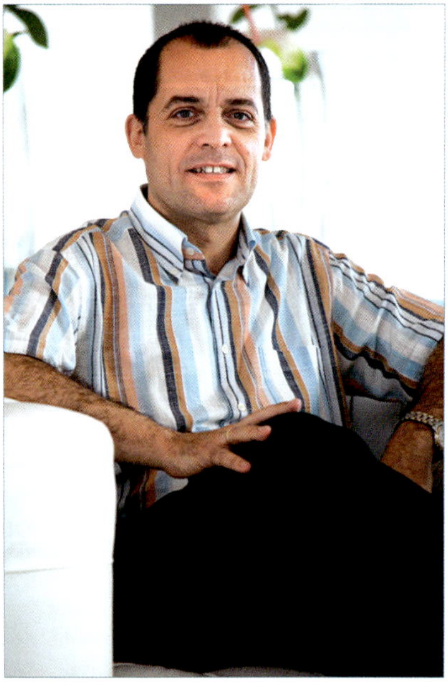

Lorenzo Fraile

Degree in Veterinary Medicine, 1992, University of Zaragoza, Spain.

PhD in Veterinary Pharmacology, 1996, University of Zaragoza.

Swine practitioner at Cargill, S.A., from November 1996 to April 1997.

Swine practitioner at Picber, S.A., from May 1997 to September 2004. This company produces 150.000 pigs by year in an integrated production system in Lleida, Spain.

He belonged to the Committee for Veterinary and Medicinal Products (CVMP) for three years (2005-2007) as a co-opted member with expertise in swine and poultry medicine. This Committee is involved in the evaluation of drugs and vaccines to be used in veterinary species at a European level. He was also a member of the Scientific Advisory Group on Antimicrobials (SAGAM) for two years (2006-2007).

From October 2004 to October 2010 he worked as a senior research scientist at the Centre de Recerca en Sanitat Animal (CReSA) in Barcelona, Spain.

He has been professor at the University of Lleida, Spain, since October 2010.

ACADEMIC EXPERIENCE

Supervisor of four doctoral theses in the field of PCV2 epidemiology (2009), veterinary immunology (2012), clinical biochemistry (2013) and pharmacology (2015). He is currently supervising three more theses.

He taught clinical pharmacology and swine pathology to veterinary students of the Autonomous University of Barcelona from 2002 to 2010.

Since 2005 he has been teaching therapeutics and clinical trial design as part of a master's degree programme in swine health and production.

AREAS OF TECHNICAL EXPERTISE

Pharmacokinetics, pharmacodynamics and PK/PD models of antibiotics and non-steroidal anti-inflammatory drugs for livestock species.

Clinical pharmacology in livestock species, mainly focused on pig and cattle medicine.

Design of clinical trials to demonstrate the efficacy of drugs and vaccines for livestock.

Design of epidemiological studies to determine the prevalence and risk factors of livestock diseases.

PUBLICATIONS AND CONFERENCES

Author of 71 peer-reviewed articles and 130 communications for international and national conferences. He has also participated as a speaker in different veterinary congresses.

Preface

In this book about practical antibiotic therapy in swine medicine, I have tried to show, in a visual and practical manner and with an updated approach, the most important aspects a veterinary clinician should take into account to design appropriate antimicrobial treatments in swine herds. This work therefore provides a review of the current knowledge in the field of pharmacology, illustrated by real clinical cases. Finally, the book includes a comprehensive review of what prudent use of these essential tools to ensure our animals' health means.

I have written this book with veterinary clinicians in mind, to provide them with a useful reference tool for their daily practice. The contents are structured in a way that will allow clinicians to reflect on the reasons for administering a particular drug treatment and to carry out a self-assessment of their work.

I really hope that you will find this book useful as a continuing education tool in your daily practice.

Dr Lorenzo Fraile

Table of contents

Introduction

1

Introduction

1

General concepts

The introduction of antimicrobials in human and veterinary medicine has been one of the most relevant medical achievements in the 19th century. The first antimicrobial agent became available in the year 1930. Many new compounds have been developed since then. However, the availability of a great number of antimicrobials has not reduced the efforts made to find new uses for old drugs or develop new products that often present a broader spectrum activity. On the other hand, a significant effort has been made in the last decade to optimise antimicrobial therapy (Scaglione, 2002).

The principles of antimicrobial therapy, including the design of rational dosing regimens, are based on a therapeutic triangle which includes the relations between the bacteria responsible for the infection, the sick animal and the drug used to treat the infection (Fig. 1). The first question that should be answered is whether antimicrobial therapy is really necessary. The objective of this book is not to make a detailed review of the clinical criteria that veterinary surgeons should follow in order to decide whether to use an antimicrobial or not. However, these criteria will be revised in each pathological entity throughout the book.

The objective of antimicrobial therapy is to provide an effective drug to destroy microorganisms and obtain clinical recovery from the infection in the affected animals. It is essential to reach both these objectives with dosing regimens that significantly reduce the probability of generating resistant microorganisms. The key questions that should be answered before applying any therapeutic regimen are what drug should be used, what dose should be administered, how often and how long for.

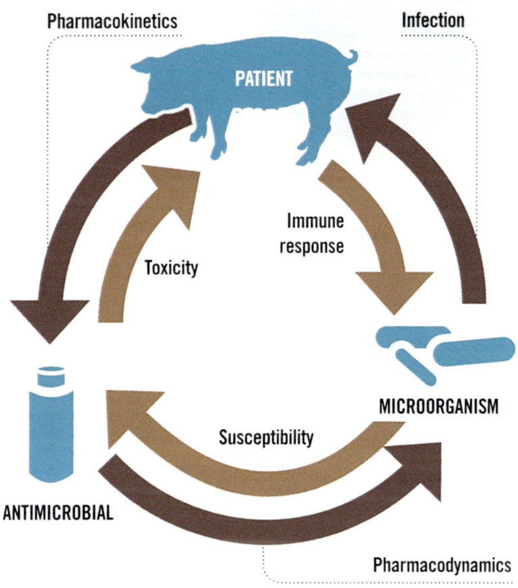

Figure 1

In order to choose a drug as well as its dose, the clinician must carefully balance the desired effects and the adverse effects of the selected agent. The key objective of the therapy is to provide a drug concentration that remains effective at the site of infection for a sufficient period of time to achieve both clinical and bacteriological recovery, avoiding at the same time the appearance of undesired effects as much as possible. Examples of undesired effects are drug toxicity in the treated animal, the development of microbial resistances to the administered drug and, in production animals, the presence of drug residues in edible tissues at levels higher than those tolerated (Lees, 2002).

Other factors that the clinician should consider when choosing an antimicrobial agent are animal welfare and the economic cost of the treatment. For example, the drug of choice may be very expensive or, in the case of a drug that is eliminated rapidly, may involve the administration of several doses per day, which would cause pain to the animal and would not be feasible from the point of view of husbandry practices in this species.

To summarise, the choice of an antimicrobial and the design of a rational dosing regimen depends on the knowledge of the microorganism that causes the disease (clinical experience or isolation), the action of the drug on the microorganism (pharmacodynamics), the action of the drug on the animal treated (toxicity), the availability of the drug in this particular animal (pharmacokinetics) together with other considerations such as the appearance of antimicrobial resistance, animal welfare and the economic cost of the treatment. All these points will be addressed throughout the book, focusing on those practical aspects that practitioners may find most interesting in their daily practice (Goodmand and Gillman, 2006).

Pharmacokinetics (PK)

The objective of administrating antimicrobials to animals is to obtain concentrations at the site of action that are appropriate to achieve the desired therapeutic effect, but not high enough to cause toxic reactions.

Pharmacokinetics is the science that describes, by means of mathematical concepts, the kinetics of these molecules when they are introduced in the organism and define a pattern of the ADME processes (absorption, distribution, metabolism and excretion) that control the availability of those substances. Good knowledge of these processes (ADME) and their mathematical quantification are therefore critical to understand the pharmacological action of antimicrobials correctly. An comprehensive description of the ADME processes can be found in excellent bibliographical reviews, as well as in books about basic pharmacology (Rowland, 1995; Baggot, 2001; Martín-Jiménez, 2002). This book about practical antibiotherapy only includes the basic pharmacokinetic concepts so they can be applied in the design of appropriate dosing regimens to treat the pathological entities (pneumonia, enteritis, etc.) that will be objects of study.

The usefulness of pharmacokinetic studies is based on assuming that the analysis of a series of plasma (or other tissues) concentrations of a drug, obtained after its administration, reflects the physiological mechanisms that lead to these concentrations. Once these processes are characterised by parameters, the latter can be used to make predictions about the concentration of antimicrobials for specific doses and thus to design the dosage regimens necessary to obtain the concentrations associated with the pharmacological effect (Baggot, 2001).

When it is necessary to describe the pharmacokinetics of a product for the first time, it is administered intravenously in the species that is the object of the study, since these mathematical models require knowing the evolution of the drug concentration after its administration in a tissue from which samples can easily be taken. Logically, the tissue that can most easily be sampled serially is the blood. The blood concentration data obtained are then adjusted by means of a nonlinear regression analysis to a polyexponential equation of the form:

$$C = \sum_{i=1}^{n} C_i \times e^{(-\lambda_i \times t)}$$

Equation 1

where C represents the blood concentration of antimicrobial at time t, C_i is the coefficient of the ith exponential term and λ_i is the exponent of the ith exponential term. This equation allows the prediction of the blood concentration of a pharmacological product at any time t after its administration. These mathematical models are based on the assumption that the kinetics of the drug are linear, that is to say, that the speed at which an antimicrobial is eliminated from the organism is directly proportional to the remaining amount in it (**equation 2**). Pharmacological products (especially antimicrobials) that show a non-linear behaviour in their kinetics are not usually used (Prescott, 2000).

$$d\,(\text{concentration})/dt = k \times \text{concentration}$$

Equation 2

K: Proportionality constant.

Figure 2 shows the evolution of the concentrations of danofloxacin administered at a dose of 1.25 mg/kg live weight by intravenous and intramuscular route in pigs, as well as its adjustment to the polyexponential equation previously mentioned.

The number of exponents necessary to describe the blood concentration curves of the antimicrobial is usually determined by applying the Akaike Information Criterion (AIC) (Yamaoka, 1978). The most important pharmacokinetic parameters are calculated according to the classical equations associated with compartmental analysis (Gibaldi, 1982). It should be taken into account that these parameters do

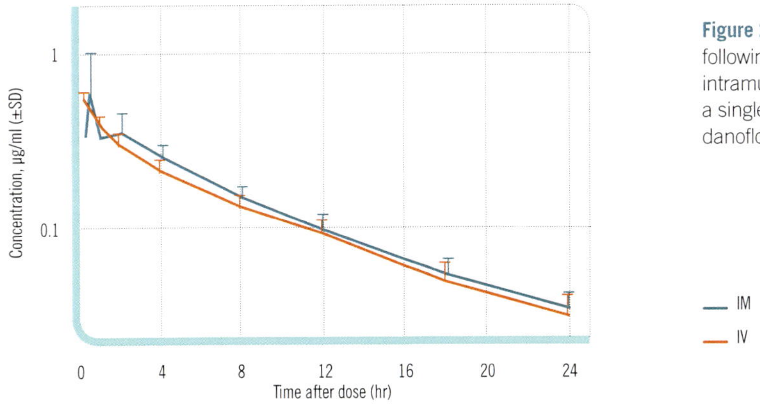

Figure 2. Plasma concentration following the intravenous or intramuscular administration of a single dose of 1.25 mg/kg of danofloxacin in pigs.

not have a full physiological meaning since they are obtained, as previously explained, by means of a mathematical adjustment of the blood or plasma concentrations of the drug.

The essential pharmacokinetic parameters that must be known to design appropriate dosing regimens or correctly interpret the information provided by pharmaceutical companies about antimicrobials are described next.

Pharmacokinetic parameters

PLASMA CLEARANCE (CL)

It is defined as the volume of blood that is cleared of a substance for each unit of time and for each kilogram of live weight (its units are ml/min/kg) and it is a direct measurement of the ability of an animal to eliminate an endogenous product or a product administered exogenously (e.g. an antimicrobial). It is the most important pharmacokinetic parameter, as it is one of the three parameters that determine the dosing regimen or maintenance dose (Toutain, 2004):

Dosing regimen (quantity of antimicrobial per unit of time) = (CL x Css)/F

Css: Steady blood concentration of the drug (steady state) that allows the desired effect. In the case of an antimicrobial, the clinical response may be an improvement of the clinical signs associated with the infection. This point will be extensively addressed in the section about pharmacodynamics.
F: Bioavailability. This parameter ranges from 0 to 1. The bioavailable dose of a product is the real amount of drug that reaches the systemic circulation (it is therefore "available" to perform its action) when a formulation is administered by extravascular route. This means that if a drug is administered orally and its bioavailability is 1, it is completely absorbed.

VOLUME OF DISTRIBUTION (VD)

It is defined as the constant of proportionality between plasma concentration and the amount of an antimicrobial in the organism. This parameter is not directly related to the distribution of the drug in specific physiological compartments. This means that a high volume of distribution does not necessarily imply that the drug is widely distributed throughout the organism, since it could show tropism for a specific organ. Thus, the volume of distribution of a drug can be much higher than the total body water volume (Toutain, 2004).

In our case, we are going to mention the volume of distribution at steady state (Vss), which is the most interesting for its clinical application. It is defined as the constant of proportionality between the amount of drug at steady state (state at which the desired concentration has been obtained and is maintained constant) and the plasma concentration at this time.

Vss = Amount of drug at steady state / Css

HALF-LIFE ($T_{1/2}$)

After the intravenous administration of a drug, the half-life is the time required for the plasma concentration to be reduced to half after the distribution equilibrium has been reached. This means that this parameter is calculated when the decrease in the plasma concentration is only due to the elimination process. This parameter is not very relevant from a practical point of view (Toutain, 2004). Nevertheless, it is interesting to point out that, after the administration of multiple doses of a drug, steady state is reached after 3 to 5 half-lives have gone by. So, for a drug with a 12-hour half-life, steady state will be reached after the second or third day of administration (30–60 hours). For this reason, for drugs with very long half-lives (> 24 hours), the use of a loading dose (explained further on) to rapidly reach steady state can be interesting and justifiable.

AREA UNDER THE CURVE (AUC)

It is the area delimited by plasma concentrations according to time. In Figure 3, it is represented by the shaded area. From a mathematical point of view, it is the integral of the concentration-time function between the points for which we want to calculate it (Toutain, 2004[d]).

A parameter that should be taken into account, although it is not derived from the pharmacokinetic adjustment of the plasma concentration data in function of time, is the binding to plasma proteins. All the drugs bind, to a greater or lesser extent, to plasma proteins in a reversible way. Only the unbound fraction (not bound to the proteins) has a pharmacological effect. This parameter must therefore be known for each antimicrobial and in each domestic species (it is species-specific). However, this parameter is not usually very relevant from a practical point of view because the binding of most antimicrobials to plasma proteins is quite low. Nevertheless, this value should be taken into account when establishing the dosing regimen in case binding to plasma proteins is high for a certain drug or species (Craig, 1989).

The physiochemical characteristics of the different groups of antimicrobials will not be seen in detail in this book. However, their main characteristics are summarised in Table 1 (at the end of this chapter), which highlights the differences between them. The next chapters of this book will analyse the physicochemical characteristics that are important for the selection of an antimicrobial for a given pathological condition.

Equation 1 allows us to predict the blood concentration of a drug after its administration, but it does not allow us to know the concentrations in the other tissues of the organism at the same kinetic times. It is a mistake to assume that tissue concentration is the same as plasma concentration at any kinetic time. On the other hand, it is important to know the tissue concentration since it is the concentration of antimicrobial in the target organ/s. It is essential to have data from a pharmacokinetic study in tissues (tissue kinetic study) if we want to know the evolution of the antimicrobial concentrations in these tissues. The most practical study that could be carried out is a tissue kinetic study after steady state has been reached. This study allows the calculation of the partition coefficient (P), which is defined as the quotient between the tissue concentration at steady state (Ctss) and the plasma concentration of the antimicrobial at steady state (Cpss). The value of P gives information about the degree of accumulation of the antimicrobials in the tissues of interest and it is very useful to evaluate the potential effectiveness of antibacterial treatments in specific organs or tissues (Sánchez-Rubio, 1999).

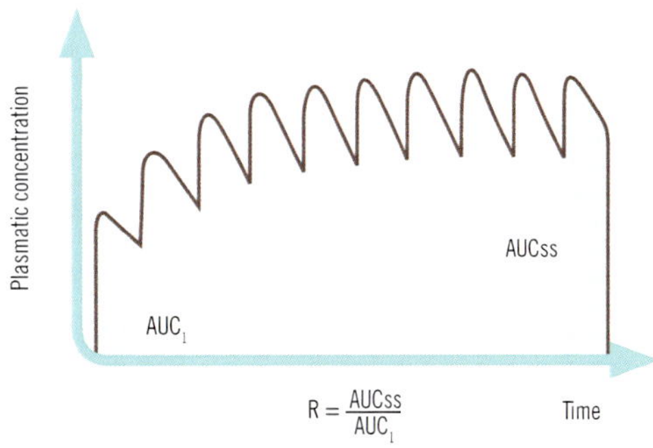

Figure 3

AUC: area under the curve after administration of the first oral dose.
AUCss: area under the curve after reaching the steady state.
R: index of accumulation = AUCss/AUC ratio.

An example of this type of study, carried out in pigs for danofloxacin, can be seen in Figure 4. These studies allow us to know the ratio between tissue concentration and blood concentration.

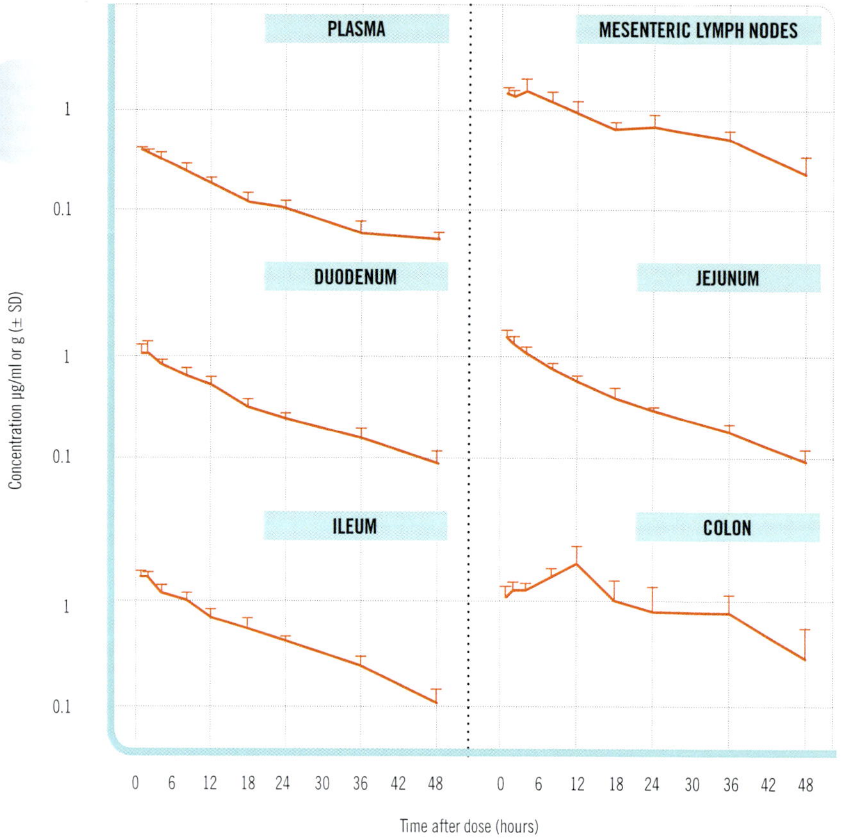

Figure 4. Plasma and enteric tissue concentrations following a single intramuscular administration of a dose of 1.25 mg/kg danofloxacin in pigs.

It can be claimed that the treatment of a typical infection process must last between 3 and 7 days in order to reach the therapeutic objective. Although the intravenous route is compulsory to characterise the pharmacokinetic properties of a drug, it cannot be used in veterinary medicine as a practical route of administration, especially when large populations are treated. That is why the most commonly used route of administration in production animals is the oral route, by adding the product to drinking water and/or feed. In large populations, the intramuscular route is used to treat diseases in a small subpopulation (usually the animals with the most severe clinical picture). In the case of companion animals, oral administration (tablets) is also more convenient than the intramuscular route.

Treatment with an antimicrobial will be very effective if the concentration of the pharmacological product necessary in the blood and/or other tissues is reached. The repeated administration of multiple doses of a drug at regular intervals that are shorter than 5 half-lives leads to the accumulation of the drug until reaching steady state. This steady state is reached when 3 to 5 half-lives have gone by. In Figure 5, we can see how steady state is reached for oxytetracycline after its administration at a dose of 20 mg/kg live weight in pig feed (Del Castillo, 1998).

When an antimicrobial is administered in feed, the plasma concentration shows a fluctuation throughout the day from a minimum concentration (Cmin) to a maximum concentration (Cmax), which perfectly reflects the feeding pattern of the animals. Figure 6 shows how the plasma concentration of chlortetracycline added to pig feed at a dose of 220 ppm varies throughout the day. It can also be seen that the average plasma concentration at steady state is 0.32 µg/ml.

Finally, an immediate therapeutic action may be required. In this case, it may be necessary to administer a dose with which the concentration at steady state is obtained directly, without

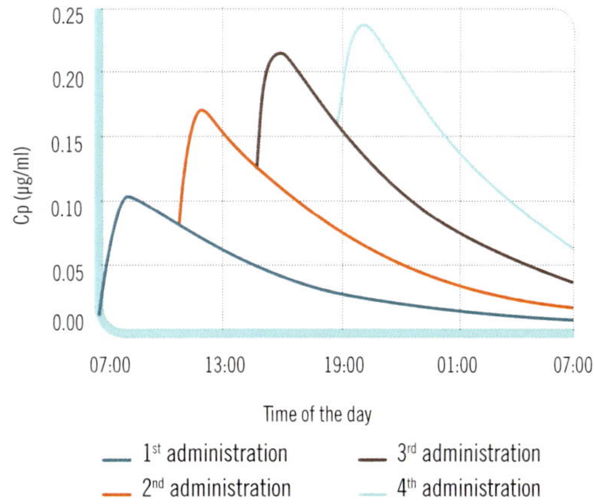

Figure 5. Simulation of the steady state for oxytetracycline after administering a dose of 20 mg/kg in the pig's feed.

having to wait for 5 half-lives. This is what is known as loading dose and it is calculated in the following way:

$$\text{Loading dose} = (Css \times Vd)/F$$

Css: Steady blood concentration of the drug (steady state) that allows the desired clinical response. **Vd**: Volume of distribution at steady state.
F: Bioavailability. This parameter ranges from 0 to 1. The bioavailable dose of a product is the real amount of drug that reaches the systemic circulation (it is therefore "available" to perform its action) when a formulation is administered by extravascular route. This means that if is a drug is administered orally and its bioavailability is 1, it is completely absorbed.

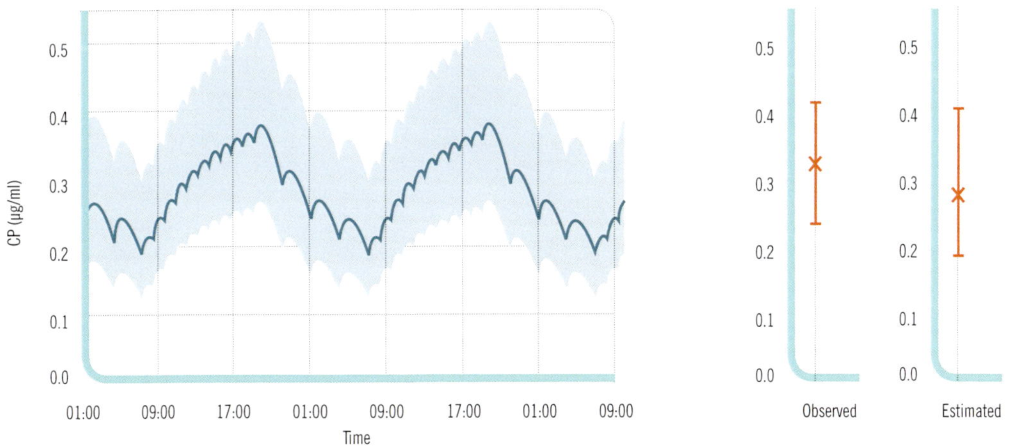

Figure 6. Observed and estimated plasmatic concentrations after adding 220 ppm to the pig's feed throughout the day (Andrews, 1988). The mean observed and estimated concentrations in steady state are 0.32 and 0.29 µg/ml, respectively.

The administration of a loading dose for drugs that are widely and slowly distributed raises the risk of an overdose caused by excessively high transitory concentrations.

Pharmacokinetics at population level

The pharmacokinetic parameters for an antimicrobial are calculated using studies that are carried out with a very limited number of animals (e.g. 10–20 pigs per administration route). It is assumed that the average values obtained are a good estimation of the values for the population (e.g. the whole world's pig population). However, there could be subpopulations (e.g. specific breeds of pigs) in which the estimation may not be correct and pharmacokinetic parameters are used incorrectly. One of the antimicrobials (valnemulin) that has recently been authorised in Europe for the control of swine dysentery cannot be used in pig breeds from Scandinavian origin because these animals cannot metabolise this antimicrobial effectively, since they have a very low concentration of the main enzyme responsible for its metabolism (a cytochrome at the level of the liver microsomes). This peculiarity was discovered through the adverse reactions (intoxication) shown by pigs of this origin after being treated with valnemulin. Such cases highlight the importance for clinicians to declare any adverse reaction to the administration of drugs to their national pharmacovigilance network.

Finally, the same technology regarding population pharmacokinetics as in human pharmacology is starting to be developed in veterinary therapeutics (Martín-Jiménez, 1997). Theoretically, this technology will allow us to design dosing regimens that are adapted to the pharmacokinetic characteristics of each patient. However, this approach is not currently applied under practical conditions in veterinary medicine.

Factors that can modify pharmacokinetics

All the basic pharmacokinetics studies are carried out in adult animals. However, many antimicrobials are administered during the paediatric phase (when animals more frequently suffer from infectious diseases). This is a critical stage of life, given the particular vulnerability of these animals to the use of xenobiotics. The developing individual is adapting to its new environmental conditions through anatomical and physiological changes that rapidly take place. As a consequence, the immaturity of various organs involved in the disposition and elimination of drugs could alter their pharmacokinetics. This modification nearly always implies a lower capacity to eliminate xenobiotics from the organism (Fraile, 1994; Fraile, 1995). However, pigs are born with well-developed kidneys; the dosage regimen during their growth should therefore not be modified in relation to that of adults if the drug studied is essentially cleared through this organ. Short and Clarke (1984) point out, referring to penicillins, that their dosage does not require any type of adjustment from the second or third day of life in cows, goats, lambs and foals.

Amoxicillin is essentially cleared through the kidney. Thus, it is not necessary to carry out any type of adjustment in young pigs since the essential parameters (both PK and PD) that determine the dosing regimen remain constant during the development of the animal (MIC and plasma clearance). However, these basic parameters could be modified for other antimicrobials in young individuals of other species and this should be taken into account when establishing a dosing regimen.

Other factors can modify the pharmacokinetics of antimicrobials, such as pregnancy, the presence of concomitant (kidney or liver) diseases or specific physiological states (e.g. lactation). Reviewing all these factors in depth is not the objective of this book; however, they will be taken into account when studying aspects of therapeutics in the pathological conditions addressed.

Pharmacodynamics (PD)

The target of antimicrobial therapy is the microorganism responsible for the infectious disease. Its elimination from the organism will therefore be critical to cure the disease. However, these drugs do not completely eliminate a pathogen without the help of the immune system. In fact, the main objective of antimicrobial therapy is to help the natural defence mechanisms to eliminate the infectious agent (Prescott, 2000).

Pharmacodynamics describes the relationship between the time-course of the concentration of an antimicrobial in the organism and the intensity and duration of its pharmacological effects. It is important to take into account that this interaction takes place between the drug and the microorganism responsible for the infection, but it will also inexorably take place between the antimicrobial and the saprophytic flora of each individual. In this particular case, the effect that is usually measured is the inhibition of bacterial growth more than the destruction of the microorganism. The measurement of growth inhibition is carried out with in vitro microbiological techniques. These techniques allow clinicians to know the susceptibility of the microorganism to one or several antimicrobials.

The objective of this book is not to describe all the microbiological techniques that can be used to determine the pharmacodynamics of antimicrobials. Those interested in these techniques should refer to specialised references (CLSI, 2011). From a practical point of view, we should have access to the sensitivity pattern of the microorganisms to be treated to the maximum amount of antimicrobials. In any case, the techniques available allow us to define the sensitivity of a microorganism to an antimicrobial qualitatively (susceptible, intermediate or resistant) or quantitatively through different parameters:

Pharmacodynamic parameters

MINIMUM INHIBITORY CONCENTRATION (MIC)

The MIC is the lowest antimicrobial concentration that inhibits in vitro the growth of the target bacteria in specific conditions of incubation (usually after 18 to 24 hours in a culture medium at 37 °C and with a standard amount of inoculums) (Sánchez-Rubio, 1999; McKellar, 2004). These conditions are not the same as those in which bacteria grow in vivo (blood, extracellular fluid, intracellular environment, urine, milk or in the presence of pus or debris). This fact allows us to easily understand that the data obtained in vitro does not have to perfectly reflect what happens in vivo. In spite of its limitations, the MIC is the most used pharmacodynamic parameter in the case of antimicrobials (Mouton, 2005).

Not all the strains of a bacterium have the same MIC. For this reason, two criteria are used to evaluate the susceptibility of a bacterial species to an antimicrobial. They are the MIC 50 and the MIC 90 and they are defined as the lowest concentration of antimicrobial that inhibits growth of 50 % and 90 % of the total population of the target bacteria. (Figs. 7 and 8).

MINIMUM BACTERICIDAL CONCENTRATION (MBC)

The minimum bactericidal concentration is defined as the lowest concentration of antimicrobial able to reduce the initial bacterial population by 99.99 % after 24 hours of incubation at 37 °C and with a standard amount of inoculums.

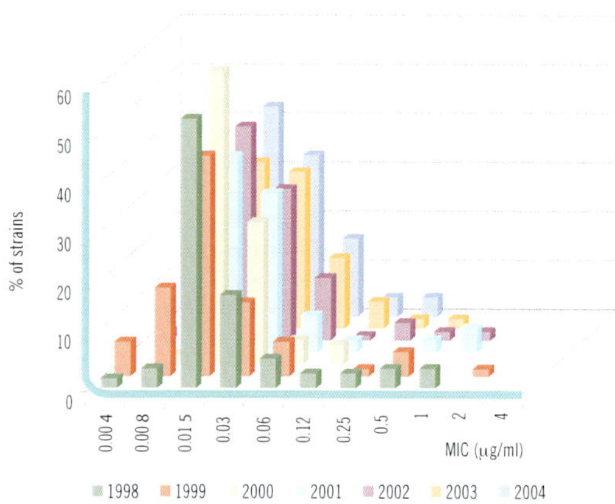

Figure 7

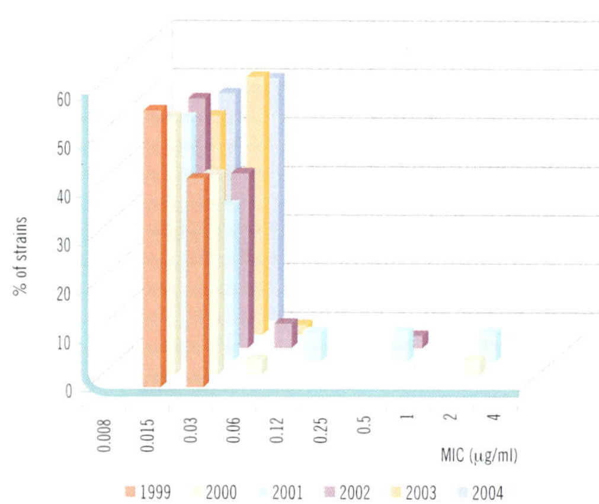

Figure 8

It has been demonstrated that the MIC and MBC for bactericidal antimicrobials are very similar; for this reason, the MIC gives a good approximation of the bactericidal activity for this type of antimicrobials. In addition, the techniques to quantify the MBC are very complicated. It is therefore easy to understand why the MIC is used as a key pharmacodynamic parameter in antibiotherapy.

Post-antimicrobial effect (PAE) and post-antimicrobial leukocyte enhancement effect (PALE)

The analysis of the susceptibility of a bacterium to an antimicrobial carried out in vitro can underestimate the activity in vivo due to the PAE and PALE.

The post-antimicrobial effect (PAE) can be defined as the growth suppression of a microorganism as a consequence of being exposed to an antimicrobial although at that time the drug is no longer at the site of action. It can be quantified as the difference between the times needed by two populations of the same bacteria, one that has never been exposed to an antimicrobial and the other that has already been exposed, to multiply their population by 10. The intensity of the effect depends on the microorganism, the drug, the concentration reached and the time of exposure. In addition, this effect is greater in vivo than in vitro (Mouton, 2005).

The drugs that show the greatest post-antimicrobial effect are macrolides, fluoroquinolones and aminoglycosides for gram-negative bacteria and β-lactams only for gram-positive bacteria (except carbapenems, which also show this effect for gram-negative bacteria). This effect can be very important since it can explain the efficacy shown by concentration-dependent antimicrobials (see next) when they are administered at very long dosing intervals.

The post-antimicrobial leukocyte enhancement effect (PALE) can be defined as the highest susceptibility to phagocytosis shown by bacteria after exposure to an antimicrobial. The drugs with a greater PAE effect tend to have a greater PALE. Obviously, this effect is not taken into account in in vitro studies and can be significant when it comes to explaining the efficacy of some dosing regimens in the treatment of certain diseases.

Utility of PK/PD models. Design of the dosing regimen. Classification of antimicrobials. Practical aspects of dosing regimen

PK/PD models

A PK/PD model is a mathematical description that provides clinically relevant information about the relation between the pharmacokinetics of a drug and its pharmacological effect. Nowadays, both microbiologists and specialists in infectious diseases believe that PK/PD models can be an appropriate tool for the design of optimum dosing regimens. However, these studies cannot substitute clinical efficacy studies although they should be complementary when it comes to designing a dosing regimen.

Obviously, all the preliminary studies about any drug must aim at defining the ideal dosing regimen for the treatment of clinical diseases. The data obtained from preclinical studies, experimental trials and clinical efficacy tests link, in various ways, the information obtained from pharmacokinetic, pharmacodynamic and toxicological studies. There are three ways of finding the most appropriate dosing regimen. These will be described next.

Design of the dosing regimen

DOSE TITRATION STUDIES

In these studies, two or more dosing regimens are applied in a group of animals using a crossover design, or in two different groups of animals using a parallel design, first in experimental infection models and then under field conditions (the disease under its "natural" conditions of expression). The result is evaluated only in relation to the clinical outcome. In this case, there is no information about the concentration levels of the antimicrobial in plasma or other tissues that could be associated with pharmacodynamic parameters. This type of procedure could be defined as a "trial and error" procedure. It is the most commonly used method historically.

STUDIES IN WHICH PHARMACOKINETIC AND PHARMACODYNAMIC INFORMATION IS "INTEGRATED"

In this case, pharmacodynamic parameters obtained in vitro (e.g. MIC) are integrated with one or more pharmacokinetic parameters (e.g. AUC). The objective is to find the most appropriate dosing regimen to obtain a steady-state plasma concentration profile with which the pharmacodynamic parameter is optimum so the selected therapeutic objective can be reached.

STUDIES IN WHICH PHARMACOKINETIC AND PHARMACODYNAMIC DATA ARE MODELISED (PK/PD MODELS)

The difference between integration (previous point) and modelisation is that in integration, the data obtained from separate studies are generally put in common. However, modelisation uses one only model that takes both pharmacokinetic and pharmacodynamic parameters into account. The most useful pharmacokinetic parameters are the AUC, Cmax and the time at which plasma concentrations exceed a previously defined pharmacodynamic threshold. The most used pharmacodynamic parameter in the case of antimicrobials, as previously explained in detail, is the MIC.

As previously said, the relation between the concentration of the antimicrobial in the tissues of the treated animal and the effect on the target bacteria is not simple. The efficacy of a treatment could depend on reaching a plasma concentration several times higher than the MIC of the pathogen (Cmax/MIC), on maintaining a plasma concentration above the MIC for a prolonged period of time (T > MIC) (Craig, 1998) or, for some drugs and pathogens, on a combination of the time of exposure to the antimicrobial and the concentration reached (AUC/MIC). If these objectives are not reached, resistant strains are more likely to appear after treatment, as will be explained in more detail further on (Blondeau, 2001). The PK/PD parameters that have been studied in depth are AUC/MIC, Cmax/MIC and T > MIC.

The relation between the AUC/MIC ratio and the efficacy of the antimicrobial treatment with fluoroquinolones has been demonstrated in an experimental model (mouse infected with gram-negative bacteria). In this case, it was observed that the mortality rate varied from 100 % to 0 % when the PK/PD parameter (AUC/MIC) varied from 0 to 100, respectively. In this particular model, the objective to be reached with a dosing regimen applied to a specific clinical case would be an AUC/MIC ratio of 100 to guarantee clinical success. This value of 100 for the AUC/MIC ratio in this particular case cannot be directly extrapolated to all treatments with fluoroquinolones in veterinary medicine.

Clinical efficacy in the case of a treatment with aminoglycosides correlates very well with the Cmax/MIC parameter. Thus, clinical efficacy in human patients treated with aminoglycosides for infections caused by gram-negative bacteria is increased by 50 to 90 % if this PK/PD parameter goes from 2 to 12 (Moore, 1987). The dosage regimen that should therefore be applied will aim at achieving a Cmax/MIC ratio of at least 12.

The T > MIC index is the PK/PD index that best correlates with efficacy in the case of amoxicillin (β-lactam antimicrobial). The recovery rate in patients with otitis media treated with this antimicrobial increased from 40 to 80 % when the T > MIC index went from 10 to 100 % of the dosing interval (Craig, 1996). However, in other studies (McKellar, 2004; McKinnon, 2004) it was shown that the steady-state concentration (Css) obtained after applying the treatment is decisive when we aim to reduce the selective pressure of resistant bacterial strains in the population. Thus, McKellar et al. (2004) proposed reconsidering the classification of β-lactam antimicrobials as depending on both concentration and time of exposure (co-dependent). To conclude, the most appropriate dosage regimen will be that which maintains a Css above the MIC for most of the dosing interval (obviously, the best would be for the whole interval) but avoids the appearance of resistant strains in the population. This objective can be reached if the Css is higher than the product 5 x MIC. For this reason, the dosage regimen can be crucial in the selection of resistant strains. The selection of resistant strains is a major challenge in veterinary medicine due to the consequences it can have regarding the availability of antimicrobials. The last part of this chapter will review antimicrobial resistance in detail.

Figures 9 and 10 show how the response changes (efficacy of the antibiotic treatment) as the pharmacokinetic-pharmacodynamic parameter varies (Mouton, 2002).

Although there are general recommendations about the PK/PD indices that best correlate with clinical efficacy for each group of antimicrobials, this does not mean that these indices are the only ones or the ones that always best predict the clinical response to a treatment. Some data available in the literature indicate that the PK/PD indices that best correlate with efficacy are the AUC/MIC ratio and the Cmax/MIC ratio for β-lactams in specific cases. The T > MIC is the index that best correlates with clinical efficacy when aminoglycosides are used in the treatment of specific diseases (Sánchez-Rubio, 1999).

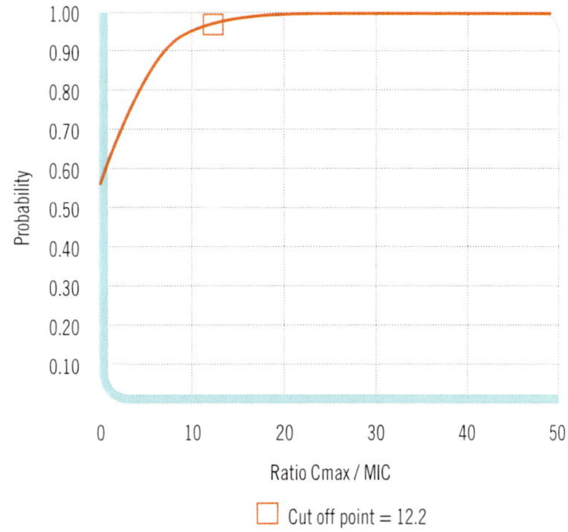

Figure 9. Probability of obtaining a clinical response in the treatment of cases of pneumonia with levofloxacin depending on the Cmax/MIC parameter. It can easily be deduced from the graph that the probability of obtaining a good clinical response is nearly 1 when the Cmax/MIC parameter is 12.2

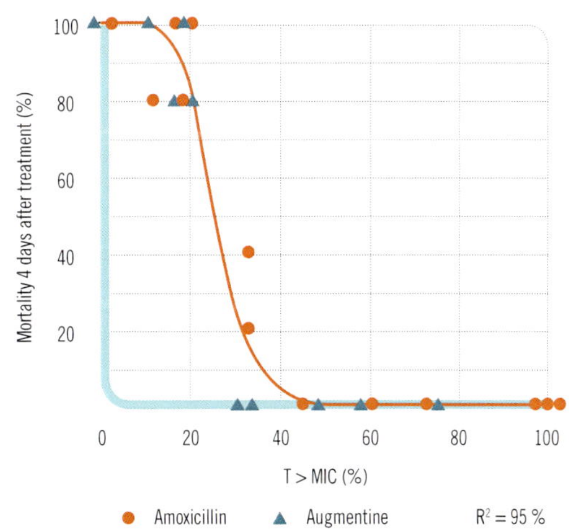

Figure 10. Relation between the T > MIC parameter obtained with various dosage regimens of amoxicillin and amoxicillin/clavulanic acid and clinical efficacy quantified as mortality in the treated patients. In this particular case, maximum clinical efficacy is obtained for these antimicrobials with a value of T > MIC = 50 %.

T > MIC: percentage of the dosing interval in which the plasma concentration is above the MIC.

Classification of antimicrobials

In general, the antimicrobials used in veterinary medicine can be divided into three groups if we take into account PK/PD parameters and their correlation with the clinical efficacy of treatments (McKellar, 2004):

1. **Concentration-dependent antimicrobials**
   They are those whose effect on microorganisms depends on their concentration (aminoglycosides and fluoroquinolones). In this case, the Cmax/MIC ratio is the PK/PD index that best correlates with clinical efficacy.
2. **Time-dependent antimicrobials**
   They are those whose effect on microorganisms depends on the time of exposure to the drug more than on its concentration, as long as it exceeds the MIC
   (β-lactams, macrolides [not azithromycin], clindamycin and vancomycin). In this case, the T > MIC is the PK/PD index that best correlates with clinical efficacy.
3. **Co-dependent antimicrobials**
   They are those whose effect on microorganisms depends as much on their concentration as on the time of exposure (glycopeptides, β-lactams if we take resistance issues into consideration and fluoroquinolones for anaerobic germs). In this case, the PK/PD index that best correlates with clinical efficacy is usually the AUC/MIC ratio.

This classification is antimicrobial and bacteria-specific. For example, marbofloxacin presents a concentration-dependent activity for some gram-negative microorganisms (e.g. *Pseudomonas* spp.), a co-dependent activity for other gram-negative germs (e.g. *Pasteurella multocida*) and a time-dependent activity for gram-positive germs (e.g. *Staphylococci*). This example clearly highlights the fact that, in order for a treatment to be clinically effective, good knowledge of the drug administered and the microorganism that needs to be eliminated is necessary to design the dosing regimen. Although it is not possible to generalise for all the cases, Table 2 shows the PK/PD parameters that can be used to predict the clinical success of treatments with antimicrobials.

In addition, it should be taken into account that much of the data used to classify those drugs come from human medicine. However, in the forthcoming chapters we will take into account the information available in veterinary medicine.

Finally, another way of classifying antimicrobials is by looking at their bacteriostatic or bactericidal action. Antimicrobials with a bacteriostatic effect would be those that only inhibit bacterial growth, so that the clinical and bacteriological resolution of the infection will depend on the animal's immune system (e.g. tetracyclines and "classic" macrolides). Conversely, bactericidal antimicrobials are able to destroy the target bacteria (e.g. β-lactams and fluoroquinolones).

Reviewing the mechanism of action of each antimicrobial is not the objective of this book. However, the mechanism of action of antimicrobials and the classification previously mentioned are shown in Figure 11 and Table 3.

Practical aspects of dosing regimen

As explained previously, the dosing regimen of any antimicrobial is established by pharmaceutical companies after carrying out many preclinical and clinical studies and described in detail in the summary of product characteristics. This dosing regimen is defined by the dose of antimicrobial to be administered, the frequency of administration (e.g. one shot-treatment or three

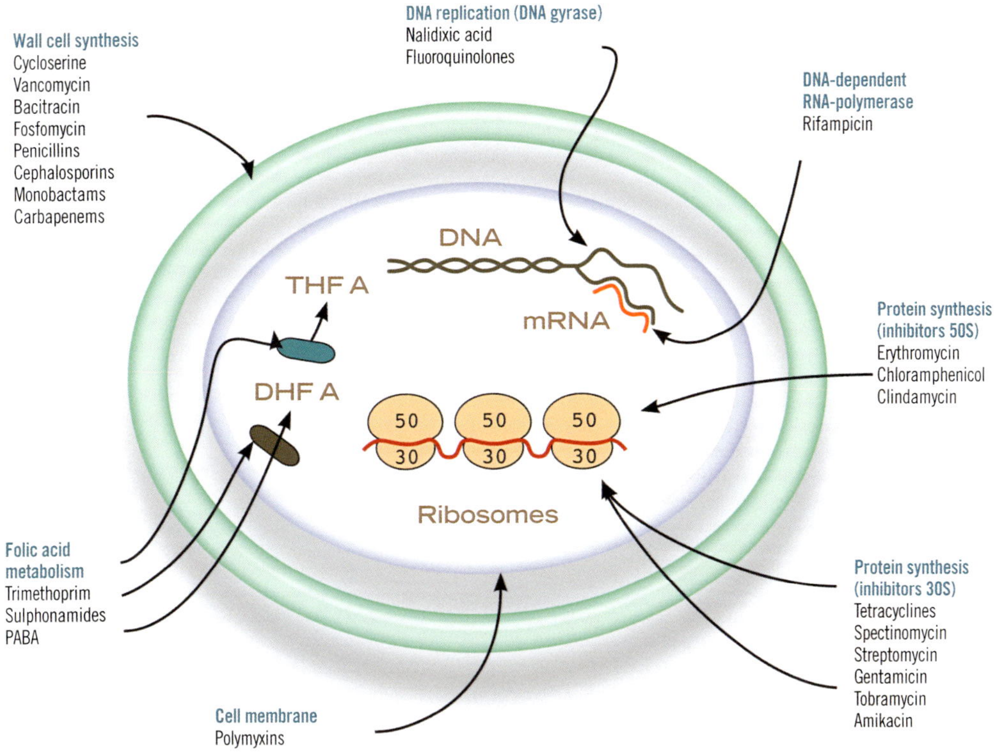

Figure 11

times by day) and the total treatment duration. For a practitioner, it is very interesting to be able to analyse the dosing regimen applied to a population of animals under field conditions. An example is thus given of how to evaluate the suitability of a dosing regimen with amoxicillin administered orally in feed at a dose of 400 ppm to treat cases of streptococcal meningitis and prevent the appearance of polyserositis (Glässer's disease) in weaning piglets.

For this antimicrobial, the T > MIC index is the PK/PD index that best correlates with efficacy. The objective is therefore to achieve a Css of 0.5 µg/ml since the MIC 90 has this value as can be seen in Table 4.

Firstly, it is necessary to know the antimicrobial dose (expressed in mg/kg) that the animal ingests daily in an *ad libitum* feeding system. The dose used in the feed was 400 ppm of amoxicillin and the amount of feed ingested by pigs with a weight between 15 and 25 kg ranges from 0.9 and 1.2 kg per day. Therefore, the daily dose that is ingested is:

Ingested daily dose (mg/kg live weight) = [ingested amount of feed (0.9-1.2 kg) x feed dosage (400 mg/kg)]/weight of the pigs (15-25 kg).

That is to say, in this case, the pigs ingest between 20-24 mg of amoxicillin/kg live weight per day.

If we calculate the daily dose that an animal should ingest by means of the following formula (see plasma clearance section):

Dose per day: [0.5 µg/ml (MIC) x 4.8 l/day/kg (CL)] / [0.136 (F)]

MIC: Minimum inhibitory concentration.
CL: Daily body clearance.
F: Bioavailability.

This means that the daily dose should be close to 18 mg/kg live weight/day. The dosage regimen that is being administered is therefore in accordance with the dosage regimen that should be administered to optimise the therapy.

Antimicrobial resistance. Clinical and microbiological breakpoints

When new antimicrobials are introduced on the market, resistant strains of microorganisms for which the active substance used to show an excellent activity can quickly appear. This process should be considered as totally natural since the antimicrobial is one more factor that determines which strain of a bacterium will be the most common in the "ecosystem". With the popularisation of molecular techniques, including typing methods, resistance mechanisms and the corresponding resistance genes have been widely documented. It is a known fact that the phenomenon of antimicrobial resistance implies a serious risk for human and animal health since it reduces the effectiveness of these drugs for the treatment of infectious diseases.

International organisations such as the World Health Organisation (WHO), the World Organisation for Animal Health (OIE) as well as institutions that regulate the commercialisation of new products in Europe (EMA) are very concerned about the development of antimicrobial resistance to human pathogens, as well as to animal pathogens, including potentially zoonotic and commensal (saprophytic flora) microorganisms. Studying antimicrobial resistance in depth is not the objective of this book, although we will revise some points that could be relevant for practitioners. All the veterinary surgeons should try to optimise dosage regimens in order to reduce the probability for resistant microorganisms to appear (FVE, 1999). If do not we take this seriously, society may see us as primarily responsible for the creation of resistant microbes and may want to limit (to the point of banning the use of whole classes of antimicrobials in veterinary medicine) the tools we can use for the treatment of infectious diseases in animals.

One of the obligations that laboratories have after starting to commercialise new antimicrobials is to monitor the appearance of resistance. This work is done through pharmacovigilance units. For this reason, it is very important that clinicians send samples of clinical cases to reference laboratories in order that this work can be carried out properly. Having this information at our disposal will help us to decide on the antimicrobial to be used in each specific clinical case.

Defining antimicrobial resistance

From a clinical point of view, resistance is defined as a state in which a patient, when infected with a specific pathogen, is treated with an adequate antimicrobial dosage and administration schedule, but the clinical criteria to consider the patient cured (at a clinical and/or a microbiological level) are not met (Turnidge, 2007). Thus, a clinical breakpoint is an MIC value that correlates with the clinical outcome and that separates those isolates that are considered as clinically susceptible or associated with a high likelihood of therapeutic success from those that are considered as clinically resistant or associated with a high likelihood of therapeutic failure.

CLINICAL BREAKPOINTS

Clinical breakpoints are calculated taking into account different criteria and are mainly influenced by pharmacokinetic/pharmacodynamic (PK/PD) parameters. PK/PD breakpoints (also referred to as concentration cut-off values) establish the probability of target attainment and thus the probability of a clinical outcome or another. They are mainly generated in animal models and then extrapolated to humans using mathematical or statistical techniques (Mouton, 2002; Turnidge, 2007). Once the PK/PD breakpoints have been established, they are adjusted to correlate MIC values with clinical outcomes. For new antimicrobial agents, these data are mainly obtained from clinical trials. For older antimicrobials, PK/PD knowledge has been scarcely applied and a process of revision of old breakpoints is currently ongoing (Kahlmeter, 2003; MacGowan, 2008).

MICROBIOLOGICAL BREAKPOINTS

From a microbiological point of view, resistance is defined as a state in which an isolate has a resistance mechanism rendering it less susceptible than other members of the same species lacking any resistance mechanism. This definition is valid irrespective of the level of resistance (i.e. low or high level of resistance) and does not necessarily correlate with clinical resistance. Isolates that are microbiologically resistant can be phenotypically recognised using the so-called epidemiological cut-off (ECOFF) value, an MIC value that separates the wild-type population from those isolates

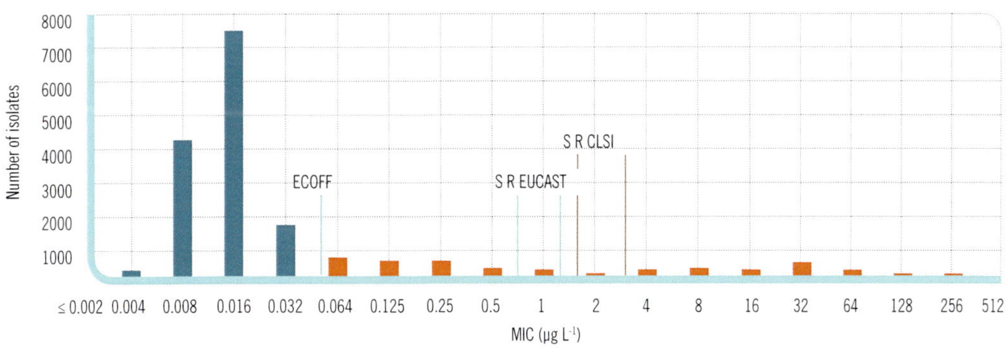

Figure 12. Ciprofloxacin MIC distribution of *Escherichia coli* isolates (http://www.eucast.org). Epidemiological cut-off (ECOFF) values and clinically susceptible (S) and resistant (R) breakpoints from CLSI and EUCAST committees are indicated. The clinically susceptible population (below the clinical susceptible breakpoint) includes part of the microbiologically resistant population (low-level resistant bacteria, presumably expressing qnr-like genes or other PMQR mechanisms or first step gyrA mutations) and the wild-type population (below the ECOFF value and presumably without resistance mechanisms). The clinically resistant population (beyond the clinical resistance breakpoint) includes isolates with high-level resistance mechanisms (most probably double-step gyrA mutants or a combination of gyrA with parC mutations).

that have developed resistance, either because of mutations or as a consequence of horizontal gene transfer, and independent of whether the level of resistance has clinical relevance (Brown, 2010). Figure 12 illustrates a wild-type population separated by the corresponding ECOFF from a bacterial population with resistance mechanisms. This figure also includes clinical breakpoints (susceptible and resistant), according to the criteria established by the two main committees defining these values: the Clinical and Laboratory Standards Institute (CLSI, 2011) and the European Committee for Antimicrobial Susceptibility Testing (EUCAST, 2011). In this table, the clinically susceptible population (below the clinically susceptible breakpoint) includes part of the microbiologically resistant population and of the wild-type population. It is important to remark that clinical breakpoints (as defined by the CLSI and EUCAST) do not try to detect the resistant organisms and are basically defined for treating patients. Bacteria may have a resistance mechanism and may be considered microbiologically resistant, and yet be susceptible from a clinical point of view.

Table 1. Classification of antimicrobials according to their hydrophylic or hydrophobic properties.

Hydrophilic drugs		**Moderately hydrophilic drugs**			**Drugs with very low hydrophily**
Strong acids	Strong bases or polar bases	Weak acids	Weak bases	Amphoteric substances	
• β-lactams: Penicillins, Cephalosporins, β-lactamase inhibitors	• Polymyxins • Aminoglycosides • Aminocyclitols	• Sulphonamides	• Macrolides • Lincosamides • Diaminopyrimidines	• Most tetracyclines	• Fluoroquinolones • Some tetracyclines: Doxycycline, Minocycline • Other drugs: Chloramphenicol, Florfenicol, Metrodinazole, Rifampicin
They do not penetrate the cell membranes or the "natural physical barriers" easily. The effective concentrations must therefore not be expected to be reached easily in the cerebrospinal fluid, milk or other transcellular fluids. However, it may be possible to reach effective concentrations in the pleura, peritoneum and joints.		In general, they pass through natural physical barriers. Penetration in the cerebrospinal fluid and in the fluids of the eye depends on the binding to plasma proteins and their hydrophily (sulphonamides and diaminopyrimidines penetrate easily while macrolides, lincosamides and tetracyclines do not). Weak bases usually concentrate in the body fluids that are more acid than plasma (milk, intracellular fluid and prostatic fluid).			Penetration in intracellular and transcellular fluids, including prostatic and bronchial secretions, is very good. Penetration in the cerebrospinal fluid is good except for tetracyclines and rifampicin.

Table 2. PK/PD parameters associated with clinical success in antimicrobial therapy.

Parameter	Antimicrobial
Cmax/MIC ratio	Aminoglycosides and fluoroquinolones.
AUC/MIC ratio	Aminoglycosides, fluoroquinolones, some macrolides (azithromycin and telithromycin) and tetracyclines.
Time above the MIC	Penicillins, cephalosporins, carbapenems, macrolides and pleuromutilins (erythromycin, clarithromycin and tiamulin) monobactems, and lincosamides.

Cmax: Maximum serum concentration.
MIC: Minimum inhibitory concentration.
AUC: Area under the curve.

Table 3. Classification of antimicrobials according to their bacteriostatic or bactericidal effect.

Action	Group	Examples
Mainly bacteriostatic	Amphenicols Macrolides Pleuromutilins Lincosamides Tetracyclines	Florfenicol Erythromycin Tiamulin Lincomycin Doxycycline, chlortetracycline
Mainly time-dependent bactericidal	Penicillins Cephalosporins	Benzylpenicillin, amoxicillin Ceftiofur
Mainly concentration-dependent bactericidal with very significant postantimicrobial action.	Aminoglycosides Fluoroquinolones	Streptomycin Marbofloxacin Enrofloxacin

Table 4. MIC population distribution of amoxicillin for *Steptococcus suis* and *Haemophilus parasuis*.

Microorganism	MIC µg/ml range	MIC_{50} µg/ml	MIC_{90} µg/ml
Streptococcus suis	0.03–1	≤ 0.03	0.06
Haemophilus parasuis	0.03–16	0.06	0.5

Treatment of respiratory diseases

2

Treatment of respiratory diseases

2

General concepts

Respiratory

The respiratory system performs many functions in the organism. Its most important function is to supply oxygen to the cardiovascular system so that it is distributed throughout the body and to eliminate carbonic anhydride from the organism. Gas exchange takes place in the pulmonary alveoli. A failure or significant disorder of gas exchange, due to pathological processes that compromise the alveolar membrane integrity or its air or blood supply, has significant consequences. In addition to gas exchange, the respiratory system performs many other functions, such as maintaining the acid-base balance, filtering and destroying emboli, metabolising bioactive substances (such as serotonin, prostaglandins and corticosteroids) and activating substances (angiotensin) (Guyton, 1996).

The anatomy of the respiratory system of a species notably differs from that of another in various aspects: shape of the upper and lower respiratory tract, extension, shape and pattern of the turbinates, branching pattern of the bronchi, anatomy of the terminal bronchioles, different distribution of the pulmonary lobes and lobules, thickness of the pleura, etc. Each anatomical variation implies a functional variation, which can have an influence on the pathogenesis of the respiratory disease in each specific species. The groups of species that have similar respiratory tracts are: 1) cattle, sheep and pigs; 2) dogs, cats, rabbits and guinea pigs; 3) horses and humans (Merck, 1991). There are also significant physiological variations among the different species. These anatomical and physiological differences essentially determine why some pathogens only affect some species (for example, *Mannheimia haemolytica* affects cattle but not swine) and why pneumonia is more frequent in some species (cattle and swine) and less in other (dogs and cats). Indeed, cattle are particularly prone to suffering respiratory diseases; among other reasons, due to retrograde drainage from the pharynx, a predisposition to pulmonary hypertension, a faster airflow rate through the respiratory tree and less efficient particle clearance from the respiratory tract (Blood and Radostits, 1992).

The functional efficacy of the respiratory system depends on its capacity to oxygenate blood and to remove carbonic anhydride from it. Any anomalies in these two functions of the respiratory system can be reflected in various ways, but the ultimate consequence will always be the lack of oxygen supply to tissues. This respiratory failure is named anoxia, or, more correctly hypoxia, and is responsible for most of the symptoms of respiratory diseases and respiratory syncope in the case of terminal diseases. Hypoxia can occur for many reasons (anaemia, congestive heart failure, etc.) but we will focus on those causes that decrease oxygen pressure in the blood going out from the lungs and that have their origin in the respiratory tract. We can mention some of these respiratory diseases such as those that oppose to the expansion of the lung (fibrosis, hydrothorax, chylothorax or haemothorax), prevent the airflow (nasal tumour, bronchiolitis, bronchoconstriction or pulmonary oedema) or thicken the air-blood interface (such as interstitial pneumonia caused by a virus or toxins and pulmonary oedema) and "fill" the pulmonary alveoli, thus partially or totally reducing their functionality (pneumonia and pulmonary oedema).

In veterinary medicine, especially in bovine and swine medicine, the most important diseases that cause respiratory failure and have their origin in the respiratory tract are the infectious diseases that thicken the blood-air interface (interstitial pneumonia) and those that fill the pulmonary alveoli with exudates due to the infectious process (pneumonia usually of bacterial origin) and the reaction (inflammation) that takes place in the organism.

The respiratory disease caused by microorganisms is often characterised by an abnormal production of secretions and exudates, and by the reduction of the capacity to expel them. A first therapeutic objective is to reduce the volume and viscosity of the secretions in order to make their expulsion easier. This can be done by controlling the infections (for example, by means of antibiotics), modifying the secretions and, when possible, improving postural drainage and removing these secretions mechanically. The therapeutic methods include modifying the inhaled air and administering expectorants, cough suppressants, bronchodilators and diuretics. Despite having quite a few therapeutic tools for the treatment of respiratory diseases caused by microorganisms in swine and bovine medicine, under practical conditions, only antimicrobials and anti-inflammatory drugs are usually used (especially NSAIDs [non-steroidal anti-inflammatory drugs]) for their therapy (Blood and Radostits, 1992).

The therapeutics of respiratory disorders must focus first on determining the aetiology of these diseases. Then, a specific therapeutic plan can be designed to solve each disease. This chapter does not aim to describe all the diseases that can affect the respiratory tract. In fact, only the respiratory diseases in which microorganisms play a key role in their pathogenesis will be addressed. In the cases of bacterial infections, an antibiotic treatment should be applied. The basic objective is to choose the most effective agent against a specific microorganism. Culturing respiratory secretions and determining sensitivity to antibiotics are the best, although not infallible, methods to design the most appropriate antibiotic treatment (Merck, 1991).

Several clinical cases of respiratory disease in pigs with acute or chronic evolution will be described. In addition, the most appropriate antibiotic therapy depending on the therapeutic objective to be achieved will be discussed in depth. Therapeutic objectives vary from the control of clinical signs to the eradication of the disease.

Penetration of the antibiotic at the site of action

In the introductory chapter, we have seen that pharmacokinetics enables us to predict the blood or plasma concentration of a drug after its administration, but it does not allow us to know the concentrations in the other tissues of the organism at the same kinetic times, unless tissue samples are also taken.

It is a mistake to assume that tissue concentration is the same as plasma concentration at any kinetic time. It is also very important to know the tissue concentration since it is the concentration of antibiotic in the target organ/s. When dealing with the treatment of an infection at lung level, it is essential to know the concentration of the drug in this organ. On many occasions, the literature mentions the partition coefficient (P), which is defined as the quotient between the tissue concentration at steady state (Ctss) and the plasma concentration of the antibiotic at steady state (Cpss). This tissue concentration is normally determined from minced lung tissue. The P value therefore gives information about the degree of accumulation of the antibiotics in the "lung" and has been used as a criterion to evaluate the potential efficacy of antibacterial treatments in this organ (Sánchez-Rubio, 1999). However, we should not take it as an absolute reference value as it does not give information as to where the drug is located exactly in the lung and in what concentration.

When dealing with the treatment of an infection in any organ (and lungs are not an exception), it is indispensable to know where the pathogen is located exactly. As can be seen in Figure 1, some microorganisms are located in the blood (septicaemia), in the interstitial fluid or even at intracellular level (Theurebatcher, 2003). It is easy to understand why it is essential to know the concentration of the drug which can be reached in the different parts that make up each organ to guarantee the success of the therapy applied in each specific case. In any case, the concentration of antimicrobial in the homogenate does not give us information about its amount in all the parts that constitute it. This concentration in the homogenate is the value used to determine the partition coefficient.

As can be seen in Figure 2, in the case of bacterial bronchopneumonia in species of veterinary interest, microorganisms are usually found adhered to the bronchial mucus and inside the alveoli, either free or inside the alveolar macrophages after their phagocytosis (Friis, 2004). It would therefore be extremely useful to know the concentration of antibiotic in bronchial secretions and in the inflammatory exudate that is inside the alveoli to predict the efficacy of an antibiotic treatment with more precision than from the plasma concentration (McKellar, 1999).

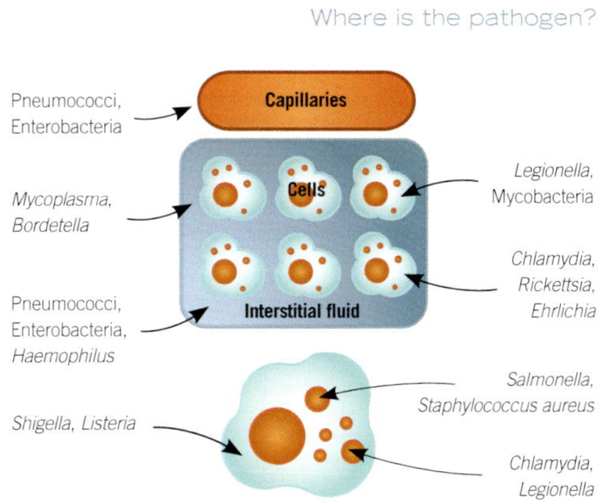

Figure 1

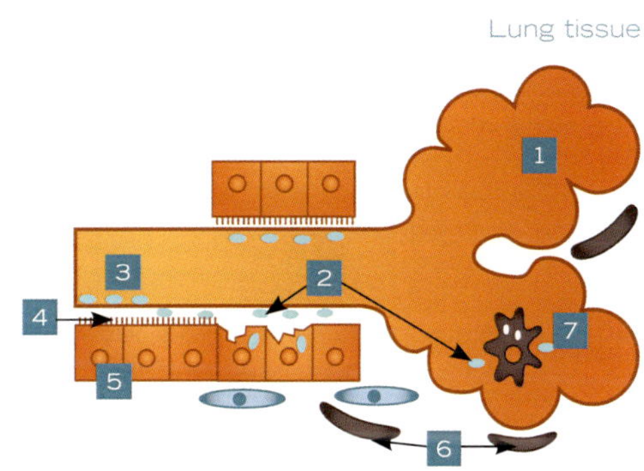

Figure 2

From a practical point of view, taking series of samples of bronchial secretions is feasible in species of veterinary interest (McKellar, 1999). However, it is impossible to take a series of samples (in the same animal) of intraalveolar inflammatory exudate. That is why systems allowing the simulation of the conditions present in intraalveolar inflammatory exudate have been designed. One of these systems involves implanting "tissue cages" in subcutaneous tissue and simulating the presence of an inflammatory process by administrating irritating substances such as carrageenan. Thus, using this approximation, it is assumed that the concentration of drug in the tissue cages is comparable to the concentration in the alveolar inflammatory exudate. This way, it is possible to determine the presence of a drug in plasma (classical kinetics), bronchial exudate (serial sampling) and inflammatory exudate by means of serial sampling in tissue cages.

Other techniques that allow the measurement of the concentration of a drug in extracellular fluid have been developed recently. One of these techniques is microdialysis (Liu, 2005). In this case, we need to find an organ for which the results of microdialysis are comparable to those obtained at lung level, but which can easily be sampled. In the case of cefpodoxime (cephalosporin used in human medicine), a study carried out in rats determined that the results obtained in the muscles could be extrapolated to the lung. However, this technique has only been used at experimental level and not in species of veterinary interest. Some papers have been published recently that describe the concentration of antibiotic in the pulmonary epithelial lining fluid (PELF) of species of veterinary interest (Giguère, 2012; Villarino, 2012). This information can be obtained through the estimation of the volume of PELF by using an urea dilution method (Conte, 1996; Rennard, 1986), whose exhaustive description is out of the scope of this book. In any case, knowing this concentration is very relevant since antimicrobial concentration in PELF may be the most relevant parameter taking into account that bacteria are usually adhered to the bronchial mucus and inside the alveoli.

Figure 3 shows the concentration of tulathromycin in PELF and plasma after the administration of 2.5 mg/kg b.w. of this drug by intramuscular route in pigs. This information can explain why this macrolide is very efficacious to treat respiratory diseases in spite of its extremely low concentration in plasma.

Finally, it is worth highlighting that, of all the antibiotics available in veterinary medicine, fluoroquinolones, macrolides and lincosamides are those that show greater intracellular penetration. In fact, in the case of macrolides, plasma concentrations do not correlate well with the efficacy observed in clinical trials, in which only the

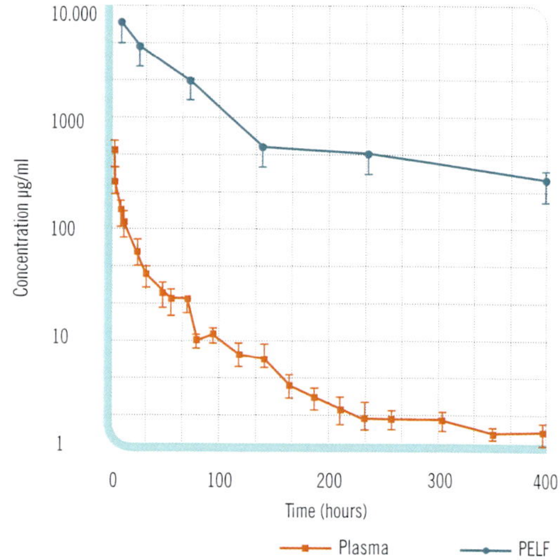

Figure 3. Mean concentration (± SE) of tulathromycin in pulmonary epithelial lining fluid (PELF) and plasma from pigs (n = 6) treated intramuscularly with this drug at a dose of 2.5 mg/kg b.w.

plasma concentration is determined, and not the concentration in the target organs. That is why drug concentrations in PELF are thought to better reflect clinical efficacy for infections caused by extracellular pathogens. High concentrations of macrolides and azalides in PELF have long been proposed as a key factor in their efficacy against respiratory pathogens in humans. The preferential activity of macrolides against extracellular pathogens in the lung has been demonstrated conclusively in mice infected with *S. pneumoniae* isolates with efflux-mediated macrolide resistance. In this study, consistent bacterial killing was observed in a lung infection model while no drug effect was seen in a thigh infection model (Maglio, 2004) These differences in the bacterial activity depending on the site are explained by the much higher drug concentrations reached in PELF compared with those obtained in plasma (Drusano, 2005).

Acute respiratory diseases

Description of the clinical case in pigs

HISTORY

- 2,500 feeder pigs of different origins.
- Age of the animals: 18 weeks of age.
- Mortality rate until the detection of the problem: 2 %.
- The animals had been vaccinated against *Mycoplasma hyopneumoniae* after entering the fattening unit with a single-dose vaccine.
- These animals had received two doses of a live vaccine against Aujeszky's disease, at weeks 8 and 12 of life.
- Herd performance until the clinical outbreak: optimum.

CLINICAL SIGNS OBSERVED

- Some animals sporadically appear with severe dyspnoea at rest, which worsens when they try to move. In addition, vomiting has been observed in some animals.
- The affected animals have fever (40.9 °C) and, without any treatment, are likely to die short (< 24 hours) after the detection of the problem.
- There are 30 dead pigs distributed in 10 pens (3 animals per pen) the day we are notified of the problem.
- There are 50 more animals showing the clinical picture on the farm.
- A necropsy is performed on the animals and the following is observed:
  - A necrohaemorrhagic pneumonia is observed in all the animals (Figs. 4 and 5).
  - In some animals, gross lesions compatible with broncho-interstitial (BIP) pneumonia are also observed (Figs. 6b and 6c) A healthy lung is also shown for comparison (Fig. 6a). Microscopic pulmonary lesions are also detected in the animals. These lesions are consistent with BIP, with attenuation and loss of the bronchiolar epithelium, mononuclear (lymphocyte and plasma cells) infiltration in the lamina propria of the bronchioli and presence of macrophages and lymphocytes within the alveoli surrounding affected bronchi; sometimes, such inflammation affects the lung interstitium. The bronchus-associated lymphoid tissue was occasionally hyperplastic (Figs. 7c and 7d). Microscopic images of healthy lungs are included for comparison (Figs. 7a and 7b).

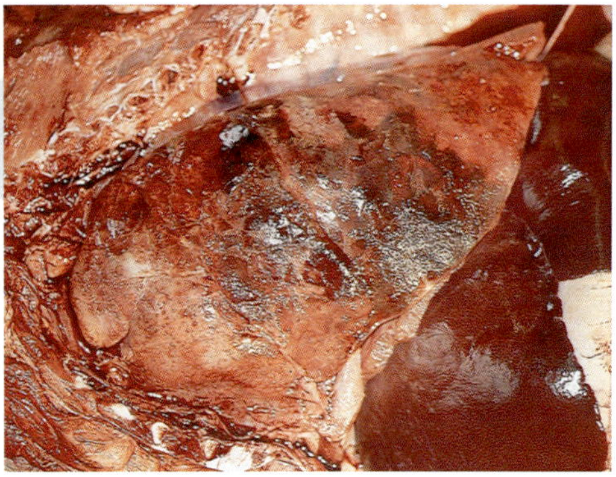

Figure 4

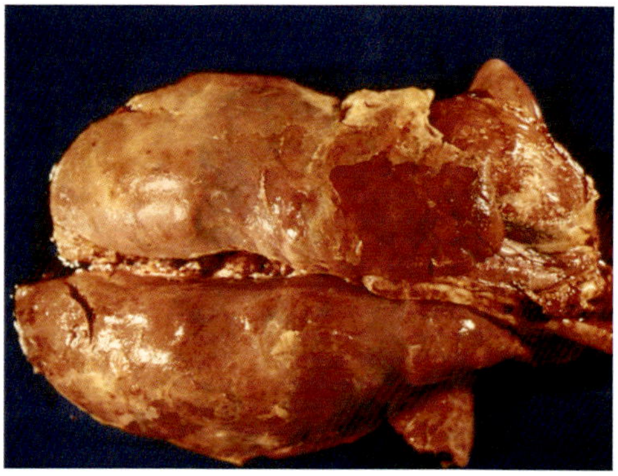

Figure 5

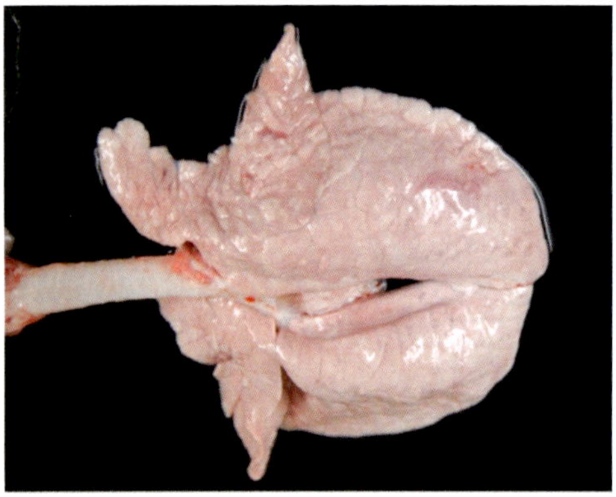

Figure 6a

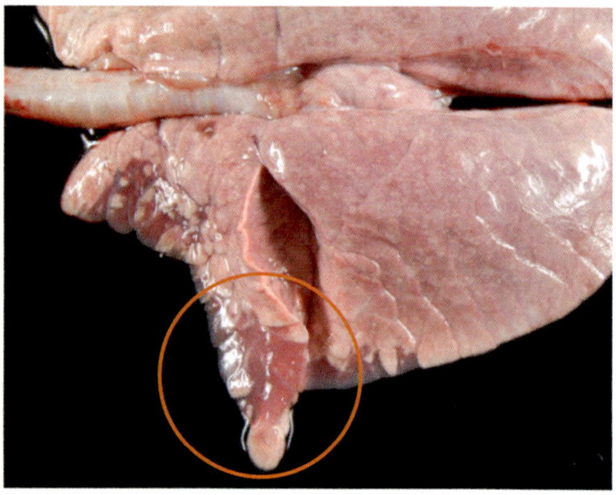

Figure 6b

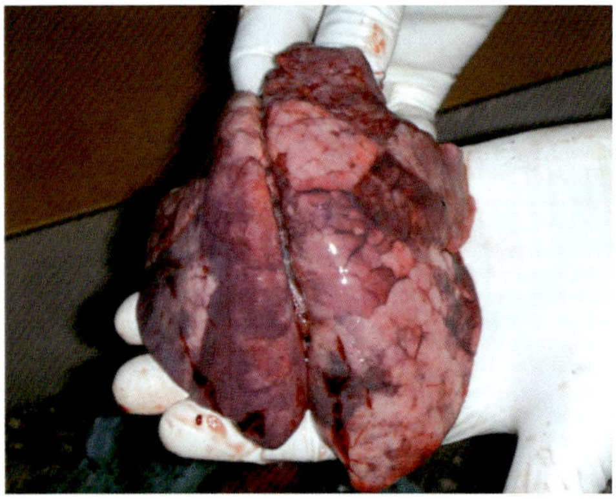

Figure 6c

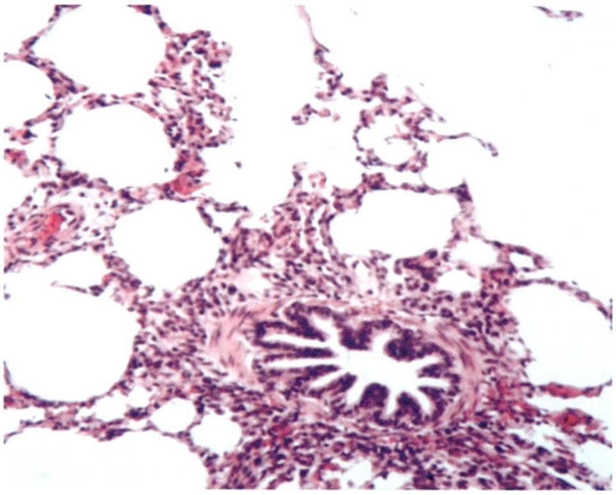

Figure 7a

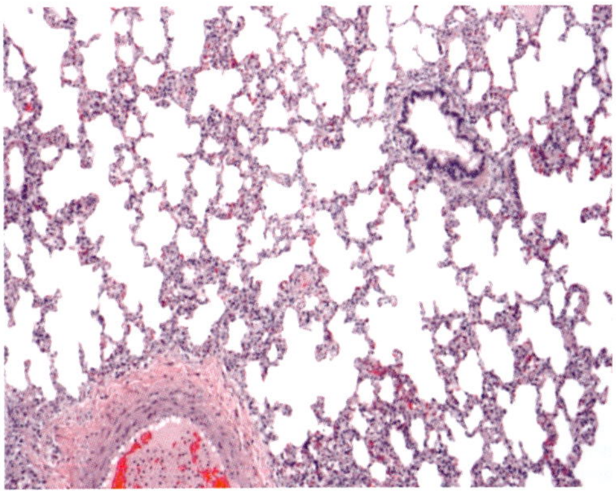

Figure 7b

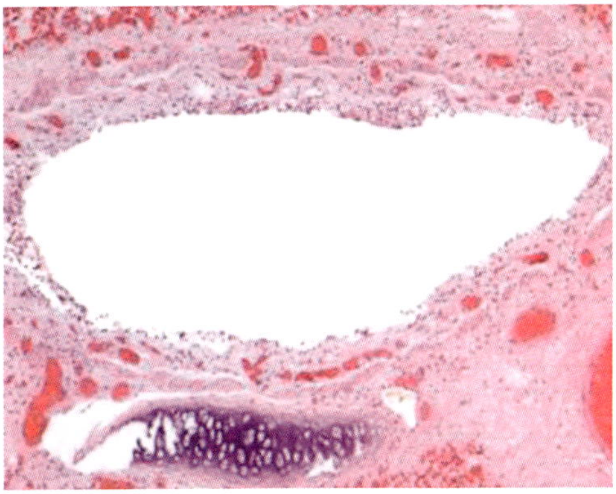

Figure 7c

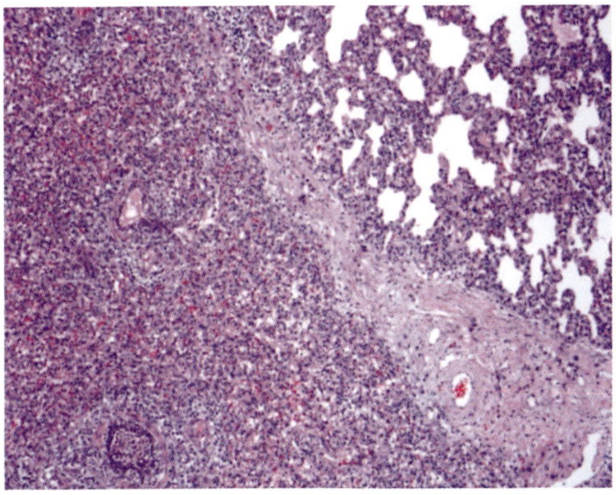

Figure 7d

PRESUMPTIVE DIAGNOSIS

- Acute outbreak of swine pleuropneumonia.
- The question that must be answered is the following: is there also a recirculation of the swine influenza virus?

Initial treatment

SYMPTOMATIC

- Acetylsalicylic acid was administered at a dose of 50 mg of active ingredient/kg live weight/day through drinking water.

AETIOLOGIC

- All the animals were vaccinated with a swine influenza virus vaccine by intramuscular route, according to the recommendations of the manufacturer.
- An antibiotic should be administered to control this bacterial infection. This point will be discussed in depth further on.
- Aerial disinfection was performed according to the recommendations of the product's manufacturer for 4 consecutive days.

BRIEF DESCRIPTION OF SWINE PLEUROPNEUMONIA

Swine pleuropneumonia, whose aetiological agent is *Actinobacillus pleuropneumoniae*, is responsible for significant economic losses in the swine industry due to its high mortality rates and the costs of the treatment of this respiratory disease.

This disease can manifest in several ways. In the hyperacute form, pleuropneumonia manifests with a temperature of up to 41.5 °C, apathy and anorexia. The animals affected by this clinical presentation have a high mortality rate. In the acute form, the affected animals' temperature reaches values between 40.5-41.0 °C and animals show clinical signs of a respiratory disease with dyspnoea, cough and anorexia. If they recover from the disease, relapses are likely to occur on the affected farms due to the fact that the microorganism has not been eliminated from the affected animals.

This microorganism is a primary pathogen and can cause a respiratory disease by itself. However, in field conditions, it can also be found associated with a recirculation of the swine influenza virus or as part of the porcine respiratory disease complex (Fraile, 2010). The porcine respiratory disease complex will be dealt with in the section about chronic respiratory diseases.

Critical review of the treatment

SYMPTOMATIC

These respiratory diseases are usually accompanied by a high temperature due to the bacterial infection. In addition, the inflammation that takes place in cases of pneumonia is one of the causes of respiratory failure. Therefore, the administration of drugs that can reduce body temperature and with an anti-inflammatory activity is indicated.

The drugs that have an anti-inflammatory, antipyretic and analgesic activity are NSAIDs. In this clinical case, acetylsalicylic acid was used. It should be highlighted that the most affected animals reduce their water intake significantly. The actual amount of drug ingested will therefore be smaller than the expected amount for animals of that age and weight. As a result, if the decision is to administer substances with an antipyretic and analgesic activity in animals that show severe dyspnoea, a very high temperature and depression (most severe clinical cases), the active ingredient should be administered by parenteral route (essentially by intramuscular route) to guarantee the administration of the appropriate dose. However, we cannot forget that we are treating populations of animals and that the administration of this active ingredient through drinking water is appropriate for the animals that are not affected and those at the initial stages of the disease. It includes the great majority of the treated population if the treatment is rapidly applied.

REVACCINATION

In this clinical case, a recirculation of the swine influenza virus concomitant with infection by *Actinobacillus pleuropneumoniae* is suspected due to the clinical signs and lesions observed at lung level. This is why the veterinary practitioner should consider the possibility of including swine influenza vaccination as part of the preventive programme against respiratory diseases on this farm.

Finally, it should be highlighted that swine influenza vaccination may be essential for the resolution of the clinical case. The administration of antibiotics as the only therapeutic measure would clearly be insufficient and would lead us to believe that the antibiotic is not effective enough, either because the dosage regimen is not correct or because resistance to the selected antibiotic has appeared.

AERIAL DISINFECTION

In this clinical case, the veterinary clinician used a disinfectant that can be used with the animals on the farm to try to reduce the infection pressure in the affected pens. The microorganism is excreted oronasally in large amounts by the animals suffering from the infection and it is a source of transmission for the animals housed in the same pen. It therefore seems reasonable to use this tool as a coadjuvant of the selected therapy. Unfortunately, there is no scientific evidence of the efficacy of this measure under field conditions. Nevertheless, it is a common practice in some countries and can be taken into consideration when planning therapeutic measures in large populations (Fraile, personal communication).

Critical review of the application of antibiotics in the treatment

Need to use antibiotics

There is a generalised consensus in the literature on the need to use antibiotics when designing a therapy in clinical cases of swine actinobacillosis (Prescott, 2000). Fortunately, there are many antibiotics available that have shown to be effective for the treatment of this disease. It is possible to use antibiotics that belong to the class of quinolones (enrofloxacin, marbofloxacin and danofloxacin), β-lactam antibiotics (amoxicillin and penicillin) cephalosporins (ceftiofur and cefquinome), classic and "new" macrolides (tilmicosin, tulathromycin and tildipirosin), amphenicols (florfenicol and thiamfenicol), aminocyclitols (spectinomycin), sulphonamides (sulfadiazine) and pleuromutilins (tiamulin).

The first question that should be answered is to what animals the antibiotic should be administered by parenteral route. Obviously, these drugs should be administered to all the animals that show clinical signs compatible with the disease. In addition, given the short period of incubation of the disease as well as the high mortality rate of the affected animals, antibiotics should be administered to all the animals in the pens where mortality has been observed, even if they are clinically normal (Fig. 8). From a strictly pharmacological point of view, it may seem that this is not justified; however, it must be done given the epidemiology and the morbidity/mortality of this disease. This therapeutic approach is metaphylaxis and it is highly recommended when dealing with an APP outbreak.

Therapeutic approach

The elements that should be taken into account are the following:

1. The infection is located in the lung. More precisely, swine actinobacillosis causes necrohaemorrhagic pneumonia in the affected animals.
2. The selected dosage regimen must reach sufficient concentrations at the site of action to inhibit bacterial growth and be maintained for a sufficient period of time. In this case, the site of action will be the bronchial epithelium and the pulmonary alveoli.
3. The antibiotic should have a very fast action since the clinical picture worsens very quickly.

An antibiotic should be chosen taking into account these considerations. In this case, the first point to be analysed is that the antimicrobial must be active against *Actinobacillus pleuropneumoniae.*

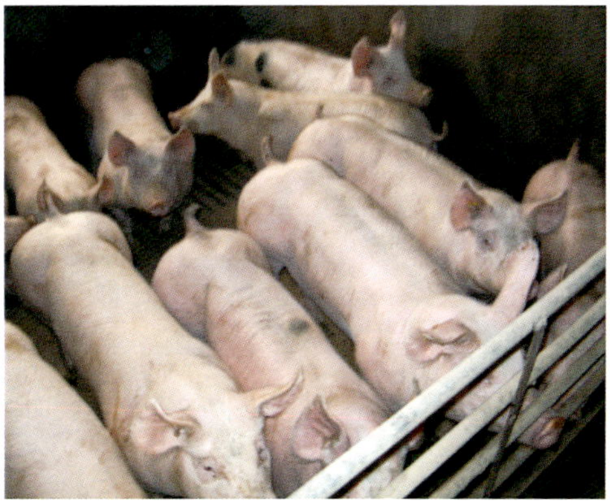

Figure 8

As seen in the first chapter, antimicrobial susceptibility against APP is usually measured with the MIC value. The table at the end of the chapter shows the MIC values for a list of antimicrobials that are potential candidates to be used in an outbreak of actinobacillosis. These studies were carried out with strains isolated in Switzerland (Table 1) and Spain (Table 2).

As explained in chapter 1, from a clinical point of view, resistance is defined as a state in which a patient, when infected with a specific pathogen, is treated with an adequate antimicrobial dosage and administration schedule, but the clinical criteria to consider the patient cured (at a clinical and/or a microbiological level) are not met (Turnidge, 2007). Thus, a clinical breakpoint is an MIC value that correlates with the clinical outcome and that separates those isolates considered as clinically susceptible or associated with a high likelihood of therapeutic success from those considered clinically resistant or that are associated with a high likelihood of therapeutic failure. On the other hand, from a microbiological point of view, resistance is defined as a state in which an isolate has a resistance mechanism rendering it less susceptible than other members of the same species lacking any resistance mechanism. This definition is valid irrespective of the level of resistance (i.e. low or high level of resistance) and does not necessarily correlate with clinical resistance. Isolates that are microbiologically resistant can be phenotypically recognised using the so-called epidemiological cut-off (ECOFF) value (Brown, 2010). Epidemiological cut-off values are given in the tables at the end of the chapter. The clinical cut-off value is usually higher than the epidemiological cut-off value (see chapter one). It is therefore easy to understand why the cut-off values given for APP in Tables 1 and 2 cannot be used as threshold values to predict the clinical efficacy of antibiotics against APP.

The second element that needs to be known is the concentration of the antimicrobial that will be reached at the site of action. In this case, the site of action is the lung and more precisely, the bronchial secretions and pulmonary alveoli. Fortunately, there is information available about the penetration of the antimicrobials that may be used to treat an APP infection in this location. This information is summarised in Table 3.

The concentration of marbofloxacin obtained in a tissue cage model (such as the one described in chapter one) is shown next as an example. This concentration is higher in the inflammatory transudate than in plasma at all kinetic times following intravenous (IV), intramuscular (IM) or oral administration (PO) of 2.5 mg/kg b.w. of the drug in pigs (Fig. 9). This observation is supported by the results obtained by Friis (2004) for another quinolone. Indeed, after the administration of an intravenous dose of 1.25 mg/kg live weight in pigs, danofloxacin reaches much higher concentrations in the lung tissue, bronchial secretions and macrophages than in plasma at the same kinetic times (Fig. 10).

The PK/PD parameters of the antimicrobials that may be used should be calculated for each clinical case in order to predict clinical efficacy in a case by case situation. Nevertheless, the probability of success can be calculated taking into account the MIC_{90} of each antibiotic, which can be found in the public domain, (Tables 1 and 2) and its pharmacokinetic properties, which can be provided by the pharmaceutical companies or found in the public domain. The different PK/PD parameters calculated for a time-dependent antibiotic (ceftiofur; Fig. 11) and a concentration-dependent antibiotic (danofloxacin; Fig. 12) are analysed as examples.

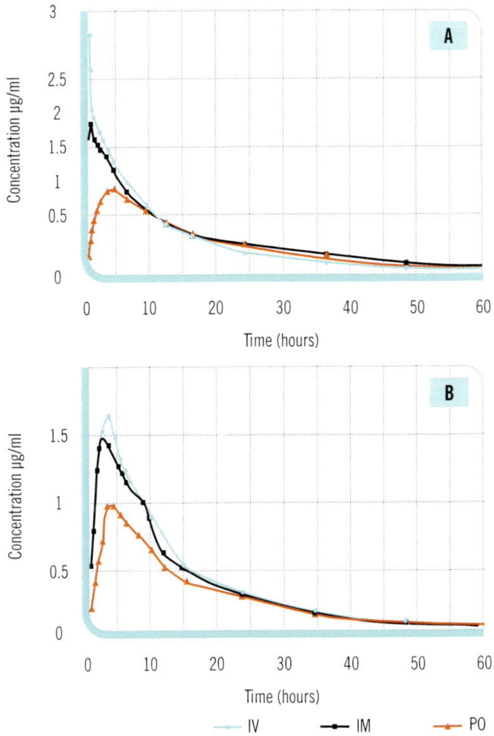

Figure 9. Plasma concentration vs. time curves (a) and tissue cage fluid (TCF) concentration vs. time curves (b) of marbofloxacin in pigs (n = 6) after IV, IM or PO administration at single dose of 2.5 mg/kg b.w.

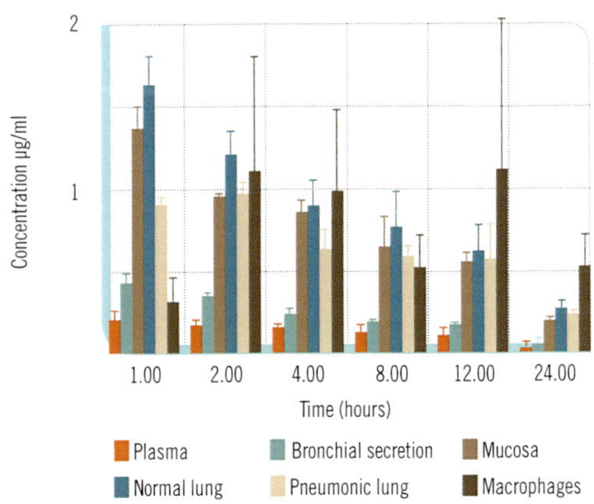

Figure 10. Tissue penetration of danofloxacin after the intravenous administration of a dose of 1.25 mg/kg live weight to healthy pigs and pigs experimentally infected with *Actinobacillus pleuropneumoniae*.

PK/PD parameter for a time-dependent antibiotic (Fig. 11)

A time-dependent antibiotic is an antibiotic with an effect on microorganisms that depends of the time of exposure to the drug more than on its concentration, as long as it exceeds the MIC. In this case the T > MIC is the PK/PD index that best correlates with clinical efficacy. As can be seen in Figure 11, the plasma concentration of ceftiofur is above the MIC_{90} for APP (0.03 µg/ml) for, at least, seven days. This treatment is therefore highly likely to achieve clinical cure of the affected animals as demonstrated in many clinical trials.

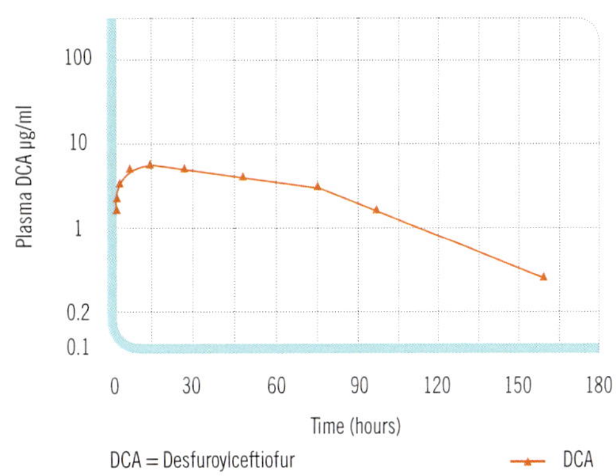

Figure 11

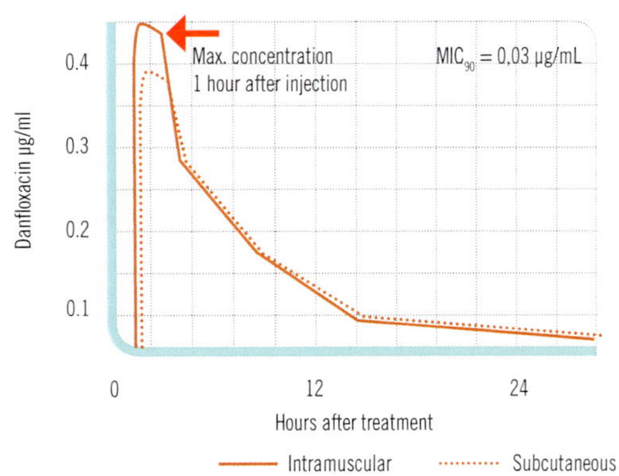

Figure 12

PK/PD parameter for a concentration-dependent antibiotic

A concentration-dependent antibiotic is an antibiotic with an effect on microorganisms that depends on its concentration. In this case, the Cmax/MIC ratio is the PK/PD index that best correlates with clinical efficacy. The value for this parameter is 3.4 (0.43/0.125) for danofloxacin and APP when it is calculated taking into account the maximum plasma concentration. This value is under the threshold value (Cmax/MIC = 10) usually accepted for quinolones. However, danofloxacin concentrates at the lung level (Fig. 13). The Cmax value in the bronchial mucosa will therefore be higher (1.2 µg/g) than the Cmax obtained in plasma (0.43 µg/ml). Considering the danofloxacin concentration observed in the bronchial mucosa and taking into account a Cmax/MIC ratio value of 10 as an indicator of efficacy, treatment of clinical cases of swine actinobacillosis with danofloxacin (Cmax /MIC = 9.6) can be expected to be effective. These results have been corroborated by clinical trials in which the efficacy of the treatment with danofloxacin for this disease has been unequivocally confirmed.

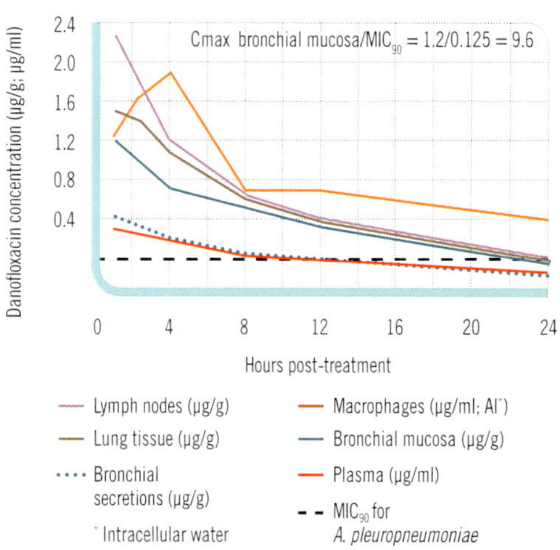

Figure 13

A summary table at the end of the chapter (Table 4) shows the likelihood of clinical success for the antimicrobials that may used for the treatment of APP infections taking into account the pharmacokinetic and pharmacodynamic information available in the public domain.

The information provided in the table is for guidance only, since every strain has its own MIC value for each antimicrobial. The PK/PD parameters of the antimicrobials that may be used should therefore be calculated for each clinical case and the result should be taken into account to optimise the therapy and choose the best antimicrobial option (Fig. 14). In addition, in order to choose an appropriate antimicrobial agent, swine practitioners should know the efficacy of the molecule (previously analysed), the current regulations on the use of antimicrobials in their country and the history of the herd.

A critical point is the selection of the most appropriate antimicrobial therapy based on the therapeutic objective we want to reach. This objective varies from the control of clinical signs to the eradication of the disease. Usually, in the case of swine actinobacillosis, the only objective is for the treatment to be effective from a clinical point of view (remission of clinical signs, improvement in performance parameters, etc.). However, it would be interesting to eradicate the microorganism in the affected animals in order to avoid recurrences and/or establish populations of pigs free from *Actinobacillus pleuropneumoniae* (APP). In this case, it will be necessary to know the penetration of the antibiotic in the tonsils (target tissue or reservoir of the bacteria). Unfortunately, there is no information available about the PK/PD parameter values that may be associated

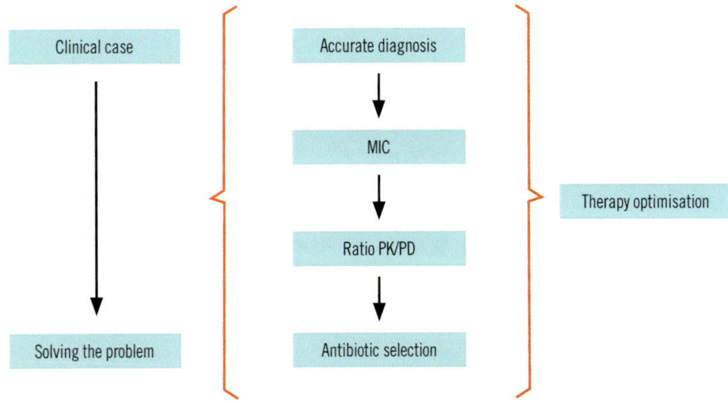

Figure 14

with the eradication of APP in infected pigs for any antimicrobial. This point is even more complicated taking into account that APP are probably located in biofilms in the tonsils. Biofilms are consortia of bacteria embedded in a self-produced polymer matrix consisting of polysaccharides, proteins and DNA (Høiby, 2010; López, 2010). The high cell density in biofilms, unlike a planktonic mode of growth, increases the absolute numbers of resistant mutants that can be selectable under antibiotic pressure. Furthermore, horizontal gene exchange is enhanced in biofilms. Whereas the mutation frequency is usually stable over time in bacteria, an increased value of this parameter has been demonstrated in bacteria growing in biofilms (García-Castillo, 2011). So-called hypermutators (= mutators) have a spontaneous mutation rate that is 10–1000 times higher than that of a wild-type strain. They are frequently recovered from chronic infections, particularly those involving the respiratory tract in humans (i.e. patients with cystic fibrosis, bronchiectasis or chronic obstructive pulmonary disease), in which biofilm formation is a feature of colonisation or infection and in which the selection of resistant mutants is high (Valderrey, 2010). A thorough revision of the treatment of bacterial infections in biofilms is out of the scope of this book but it is worth noting that some treatments used under field conditions try to eliminate bacteria located in biofilms. An example in pig medicine is applying antibiotics to eliminate *Actinobacillus pleuropneumoniae* from pig tonsil.

Chronic respiratory diseases

Description of the clinical picture

HISTORY

- The affected animals were housed in a fattening unit with space allowance for 2000 animals. The farm was free from the Aujeszky's disease virus and was positive to the porcine respiratory and reproductive syndrome (PRRS) virus.
- Percentage of death pigs until detection of the problem: 1.5 %
- The affected animals had been vaccinated against *Mycoplasma hyopneumoniae* at 7 and 21 days of age. In addition, they had received their first two vaccines against the

Aujeszky's disease virus, at 10 and 16 weeks of life.
- Herd performance until the clinical outbreak: very good.

CLINICAL SIGNS OBSERVED

- Sporadically, some animals show severe dyspnoea at rest, which worsens when they try to move.
- Age of the affected animals: between 17 and 18 weeks.
- The affected animals present with slight fever (40.0 °C) and are likely to get worse without any treatment. This worsening implies a significant growth delay. In fact, the affected batches have a low growth rate and a high feed conversion index in comparison with the results obtained in batches where the problem was not detected.
- Some animals are very depressed (Fig. 15).
- Cough is a frequent symptom in the batch of affected animals.
- The day we are notified of the problem, two pigs that belonged to two different pens die.
- There are 10 more animals with the same clinical picture on the farm.
- A necropsy is performed on two animals and the following is observed: the two necropsied animals suffered from pneumonia (Fig. 16).

The clinical picture lasts for 15 to 21 days in all the sick animals. However, the duration of the disease in a whole batch is longer than a month. This is due to the fact that new clinical cases progressively appear.

PRESUMPTIVE DIAGNOSIS

Porcine respiratory disease complex in which *Mycoplasma hyopneumoniae* seems to be involved as one of the most relevant agents together with *Pasteurella multocida*. This association used to be known as porcine enzootic pneumonia. However, nowadays it is more correct to talk about porcine respiratory disease complex.

In order to verify this initial presumptive diagnosis, the complementary studies described next were carried out:

Complementary studies

ANALYTICAL METHODS

- Serological tests were performed in order to know the serum antibodies levels of the animals against the PRRSV, Aujeszky's virus, SIV (swine influenza) and *Mycoplasma hyopneumoniae* upon their arrival at the fattening unit, when the clinical problem started and 21 days afterwards.

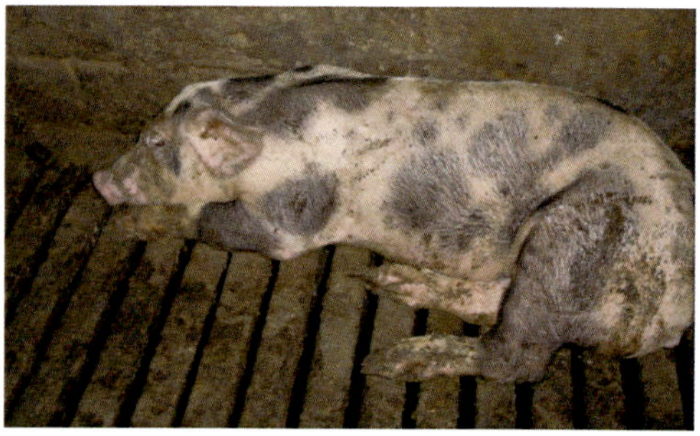

Figure 15

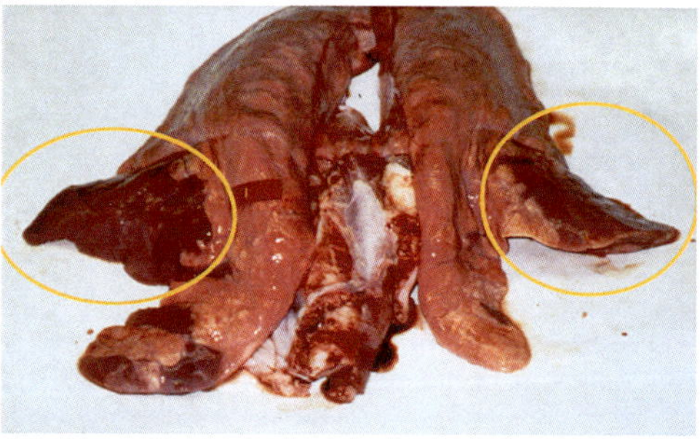

Figure 16

- Microbiological isolation of the affected lung portions.
- Pathological study of the lung.

RESULTS OF THE ANALYSIS

- The serological studies revealed seroconversion against the PRRS virus and *Mycoplasma hyopneumoniae*. These two infectious agents are therefore involved in the aetiology of the clinical case.
- *Pasteurella multocida* was isolated from all the analysed lungs.
- The lesions are compatible with an infection by *Mycoplasma hyopneumoniae*, PRRS virus and *Pasteurella multocida* as a secondary bacterial agent.

Definitive diagnosis

Porcine respiratory disease complex in which *Mycoplasma hyopneumoniae* and the PRRS virus are the primary aetiological agents and *Pasteurella multocida* plays a role as a secondary pathogen. The difference between the presumptive and definitive diagnoses highlights the importance of carrying out complementary studies when the objective is to reach a precise diagnosis in a complex in which many different microorganisms can be involved.

Brief description of the porcine respiratory disease complex

The porcine respiratory disease complex (PRDC) is a clinical condition that seems to have evolved in parallel with the modernisation of swine production. This respiratory complex is characterised clinically by the presence of dyspnoea, cough, acute depression, fever and nasal secretion, and essentially affects pigs at the fattening stage (Dee, 1996). The morbidity and mortality of this disease range from 30 % to 70 % and from 4 % to 6 %, respectively. The presence of this disease leads to an increase of $0.21 in the production costs per pig produced in a fattening unit and of $1.34 in a farrow-to-finish farm, according to a study conducted by the National Health Monitoring System (NAHMS) in the United States (Hoover, 1996).

This respiratory complex is due to the interaction of multiple factors, such as the presence of bacterial and viral microorganisms, the environment and the management system used by the farmer to raise the pigs. An "appropriate" combination of these factors can alter the defence mechanisms of the respiratory system and cause a severe respiratory disease. This disease is caused by the interaction and synergy of viral and bacterial pathogens. The viral pathogens that are most often involved are the porcine reproductive and respiratory syndrome virus (PRRSV), the swine influenza virus (SIV), the Aujeszky's disease virus (PRV) and the porcine respiratory coronavirus (PRCV). The bacterial pathogens that are most often involved in the complex are *Mycoplasma hyopneumoniae*, *Actinobacillus pleuropneumoniae*, *Bordetella bronchiseptica*, *Pasteurella multocida*, *Haemophilus parasuis*, *Streptococcus suis*, *Trueperella pyogenes*, *Salmonella cholerasuis* and *Actinobacillus suis*.

Mycoplasma hyopneumoniae colonises the respiratory tract and settles on the bronchiolar epithelium, where it causes depletion of the cilia. Affected animals present with pneumonia (in which the alveoli are filled with exudate) and there is perivascular and peribronchiolar lymphoreticular hyperplasia. This pathogen causes immunomodulation and makes it possible for other microorganisms, such as *Pasteurella multocida*, to worsen the signs of pneumonia.

It is difficult to establish a precise diagnosis of the cause of PRDC on an operation due to the multifactorial infectious aetiology that is usually involved, as occurs in the bovine respiratory syndrome, which shares many similarities with PRDC from an aetiopathogenic point of view (Desrosiers, 1997).

Many measures can be implemented to solve clinical cases of PRDC. These measures are very varied and include monitoring the environment where the animals are housed, management strategies, changes in the production flow, implementation of strategic vaccination programmes (especially against viral infectious agents such as PRRSV, PRV and SIV) and antibiotic medication (Dee, 1996; Henry and Apley, 1999). In the case of the latter, it is necessary to administer antibiotics by parenteral route and/or through drinking water.

Critical review of the treatment

SYMPTOMATIC

The same comments as for the clinical case of porcine actinobacillosis can be made in this section. However, fever is not a very relevant symptom in animals affected by PRDC (chronic cough is much more important). The use of NSAIDs in the treatment of PRDC should therefore be based on the application of strict economic criteria. This means that the symptomatic treatment should improve the final cost of production of the animals when compared with the production batches in which this support therapy is not applied. If no economic improvement is observed, this symptomatic treatment would not be justified.

AETIOLOGICAL

The aetiological treatment must aim at blocking the main aetiopathogenic mechanism in each clinical case. In this case, the respiratory complex is caused by the association of a virus (PRRSV) and two bacteria (*Mycoplasma hyopneumoniae* and *Pasteurella multocida*).

There are no antiviral drugs available for livestock in veterinary medicine that can block the multiplication of the virus. The strategy regarding the PRRS virus should therefore focus on developing active immunisation in the animals so they become "resistant" to the infection by this virus. This point is extremely controversial in porcine medicine and is beyond the objectives of this book. However, it has become a "cornerstone" in the strategies for the control of the porcine respiratory disease complex.

Two bacteria play a role in this clinical case of porcine respiratory disease. Therefore, it seems reasonable to think that antibiotic treatment is indicated either by oral or parenteral route. This point will be discussed in depth next.

CRITICAL REVIEW OF THE ADMINISTRATION OF ANTIBIOTICS IN THE TREATMENT

Need to use antibiotics

There is a generalised consensus in the literature about the need to use antibiotics in clinical cases of PRDC caused by *Mycoplasma hyopneumoniae* and *Pasteurella multocida* as bacterial pathogens (Prescott, 2000). This is the clinical case that is discussed in this section. Fortunately, there are many antibiotics available that have shown to be effective for the treatment of this disease, either alone or in combination. Many antibiotics such as quinolones (enrofloxacin, marbofloxacin and danofloxacin), "classic" macrolides (tilosin, acetylisovaleryltylosin and tilmicosin), "new" macrolides (tulathromycin), lincosamides (lincomycin) and pleuromutilins (tiamulin and valnemulin) have a relatively low MIC against *Mycoplasma hyopneumoniae*. Therefore, all these drugs would be indicated, a priori, in the treatment of porcine mycoplasmosis. On the other hand, other drugs, such as tetracyclines (chlortetracycline and oxytetracycline), have a higher MIC against this microorganism. This does not mean that they are not indicated, as it will be necessary to analyse the recommended dosage regimen for these substances. Finally, it should be highlighted that the selected drug should be active against many other bacteria (e.g. *Pasteurella multocida*) or if not, a combination of antibiotics could be used to broaden the spectrum of activity.

Therapeutic approach

The elements that should be taken into account are the following:

1. The infection is located in the lung. More precisely, the most characteristic lesion of PRDC in the affected animals is cranioventral lung consolidation.
2. The selected dosage regimen must reach concentrations at the site of action that are sufficient to inhibit bacterial growth and be maintained for a sufficient period of time. In this case, the sites of action will be the bronchial epithelium and the pulmonary alveoli.

Firstly, it should be highlighted that there is very little information available about experimental studies in which the disease is reproduced in the most similar way possible to how it occurs under field conditions. In fact, most of the experimental studies reproduce the disease by inoculating healthy animals with a homogenate from lungs with enzootic pneumonia lesions intranasally or intratracheally. The infection by *Mycoplasma hyopneumoniae* overlaps with another bacterial infection, because it is part of the challenge study, because it was a contaminant pathogen in the homogenate or because it took place as a natural infection in the animals. In studies evaluating prevention, medication starts before or right at the moment of the infection. However, in treatment studies, medication starts 10 to 28 days after the infection since in these experimental models, it is considered that lesions start to appear at that moment. In conclusion, the results obtained in different studies carried out with antibiotics are not directly comparable as it is extremely complicated to standardise experimental models in which various microorganisms are involved (Stipkovits, 2001).

The selected antibiotic should be active against *Mycoplasma hyopneumoniae* (MH) and other pathogens that may be involved. In this specific clinical case, the antibiotic should also be active against *Pasteurella multocida* (PM). Another possibility is to choose an antibiotic to control MH and another to control PM. In this case, the first characteristic that should be taken into account is that the antimicrobial must be active against MH and/or PM. As explained in the first chapter, the antimicrobial susceptibility of a bacterium is usually measured with the MIC value.

The determination of the MIC for mycoplasmas is a controversial topic. Many factors can influence the results of MIC tests involving *Mycoplasma* species of veterinary interest, including the composition and pH of the culture medium, the conditions of incubation and the preference of certain *Mycoplasma* species for agar rather than for broth media. Whether using a liquid or solid MIC assay system, it is essential, to avoid obtaining falsely low MIC results, that optimal media for growing specific mycoplasma species are used, that cultures are pure and that mycoplasma inocula are carefully standardised. The recommended viable counts for inocula are 10^3 to 10^5 ccu × ml^{-1} for liquid assays and 10^3 to 10^5 cfu per plate for the agar dilution method. The growth phase of the organisms seems to be less important, since lag phase cultures of MH have been shown to give very similar results to cultures in the logarithmic growth phase in liquid assays. Antimicrobials should be stored according to the manufacturer's recommendations and their MIC values should be determined in relation to their active base component, particularly when comparing results between laboratories. In liquid and solid MIC assays, it is important that tests are carefully controlled, with growth, sterility, pH end-point (in liquid assays) and compound solvent controls and that standard reference mycoplasmas with established antibiotic sensitivity patterns are included in each experiment. In liquid MIC assays, microdilution plates must be adequately sealed to prevent the exchange of gases between wells, which might result in false colour changes and erroneous MIC endpoints, and the reading of liquid or solid MIC tests should be carefully standardised. These factors, coupled with the lack of standardisation of MIC procedures between laboratories, have made it almost inevitable to find significant differences in results.

The tables at the end of the chapter show the MIC values of a list of antimicrobials that may be used in a coinfection with MH and PM. The epidemiolological cut-off values for antimicrobial resistance are also included. The differences between clinical and epidemiological cut-off values when the most relevant end-point is clinical cure have already been addressed.

The second element that needs to be known is the concentration of the antimicrobial that will be reached at the site of action. In this case, the site of action is the lung and more precisely, the bronchial secretions and pulmonary alveoli. Fortunately, it is possible to find information about the penetration of the antimicrobials that may be used to treat a coinfection at lung level. After taking into account the pharmacokinetic properties of the antimicrobials that may be administered, Table 3 can be used. The PK/PD parameter (T > MIC) calculated for a time-dependent antibiotic (tulathromycin; Fig. 17) is given as an example. It can be seen that the antibiotic concentration at lung level is above the MIC_{90} value for, at least, 15 days.

Finally, the probability of success (Table 8) can be calculated taking into account the MIC_{90} of each antibiotic, which can be found in the public domain (Tables 5, 6 and 7), and its pharmacokinetic properties, which can be provided by the pharmaceutical companies or found in the public domain.

The information provided in Table 8 is for guidance only, as each strain has a different MIC value for each antimicrobial. The PK/PD parameters of the antimicrobials that may be used should therefore be calculated for each clinical case and the result should be taken into account to optimise the therapy and choose the best antimicrobial option (see Fig. 14). In addition, in order to choose an appropriate antimicrobial agent, swine practitioners should know the efficacy of the molecule (previously analysed), the current regulations on the use of antimicrobials in their country and the history of the herd.

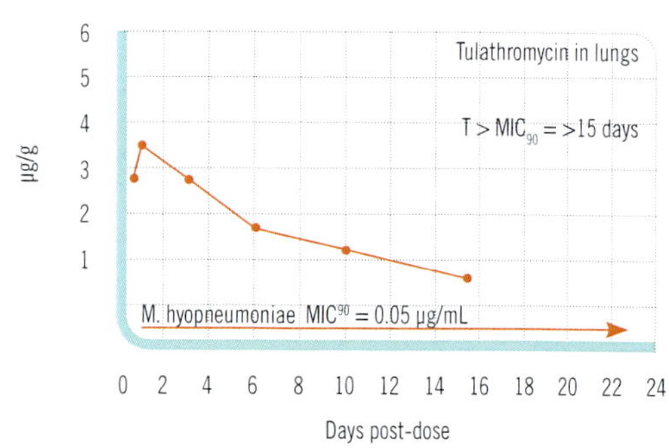

Figure 17

The results obtained in controlled studies of treatments for the prevention and treatment of enzootic pneumonia are shown in Table 9. As can be observed, efficacy is higher when the therapeutic objective is prevention when compared with the results obtained if the objective is the treatment of the disease. Nonetheless, as previously said, the results obtained in the different studies are difficult to compare due to the fact that it is extremely complicated to standardise experimental models in which several microorganisms are involved (Stipkovits, 2001) and to the intrinsic difficulty of carrying out controlled clinical trials when several microorganisms intervene in the pathogenesis of the disease. In conclusion, it is extremely important to monitor the antimicrobial treatments (mortality, morbidity, conversion index, etc.) established to control this disease in order to really evaluate their efficacy in each specific case.

Finally, several strategies have been used to eradicate *Mycoplasma hyopneumoniae* from affected farms, such as depopulation and medicating animals with a combination of antibiotics that are active against this microorganism. Unfortunately, these combinations of drugs as well as their dosage regimens were determined from clinical experience and not from PK/PD studies (Alexander, 1980; Baekbo, 1994; Lium, 1992). It is therefore impossible to carry out a comprehensive study of the therapy when its objective is to eradicate the microorganism. However, some authors claim that eradication programmes are successful in a high percentage of cases (Burch, 2006).

Table 1.1. Minimal inhibitory concentration (MIC) of 20 antimicrobial agents for 83 *A. pleuropneumoniae* isolates from pigs (Matter et al., 2007).

	Actinobacillus pleuropneumoniae **MIC (µg/ml)**																
Antimicrobial	**ATCC27090**	**0.03**	**0.06**	**0.12**	**0.25**	**0.5**	**1**	**2**	**4**	**8**	**16**	**32**	**64**	**128**	**256**	**512**	**> 512**
Cephalothin	≤ 4							79		1	3						
Celtiofur	≤ 1					83			|								
Cefquinome	≤ 1					83											
Florfenicol	≤ 1					81		1	1 |								
Enrofloxacin	≤ 0.06	75		6		1	1										
Colistin	1				26		37	17	1	2							
Erythromycin	8								16	67							
Tilmicosin	16									13	68	1	1				
Tiamulin	16									17	57	8	1				
Clindamycin	4							2	66	15							
Gentamicin	8								2	28 |	51	2					
Neomycin	> 32											21	62				
Apramycin	32										3	57	23				
Spectinomycin	64										1	2	78	1	1		
Penicillin	0.5				3	37	34	5	1		3						
Ampicillin	≤ 0.12			21	45	12	2						3				
Amoxicillin/ clavulanic acid [a]	≤ 2							82	1 |							
Tetracycline	≤ 1					76		2		3 |		2					
Sulfamethoxazole	128												3	15	32 |	22	11
Trimethoprim sulfamethoxazole [b]	≤ 0.25			79		3			| 1								

The dilution ranges tested for each antibiotic are those contained within the white area. Values above this range indicate MIC values higher than the highest concentration in the range. Values below the lowest concentration tested indicate MIC values smaller or equal to the lowest concentration in the range. CLSI resistance breakpoints are indicated with vertical black lines when available.

[a] Concentration of amoxicillin given, tested in a concentration ratio of 2:1 (amoxicillin/clavulanic acid).

[b] Concentration of trimethroprim given, tested in a concentration ratio of 1:19 (trimethoprim/sulfamethoxazole).

Table 1.2. MIC 50 % and MIC 90 % data of 20 antimicrobial agents for 83 *A. pleuropneumoniae* isolates (Matter et al., 2007).

Antimicrobial	Range	MIC (µg/ml) 50 %	MIC (µg/ml) 90 %	Percentage of resistance [a]
Cephalothin	≤ 4-16	≤4	≤4	0
Celtiofur	≤ 1	≤ 1	≤ 1	0
Cefquinome	≤ 1	≤ 1	≤ 1	n.c.
Florfenicol	≤ 1-4	≤ 1	≤ 1	0
Enrofloxacin	≤ 0.06-1	≤ 0.06	≤ 0.06	n.c.
Colistin	≤ 0.5-8	1	2	n.c.
Erythromycin	4-8	8	8	n.c.
Tilmicosin	8-32	16	16	2
Tiamulin	8-32	16	16	11
Clindamycin	2-4	4	> 4	n.c.
Gentamicin	4-16	16	16	64
Neomycin	32-32	> 32	> 32	n.c.
Apramycin	16-32	32	> 32	n.c.
Spectinomycin	16-128	64	64	n.c.
Penicillin	0.25-8	1	2	4
Ampicillin	≤ 0.25-32	0.25	0.5	4
Amoxicillin/clavulanic acid [a]	2-4	2	2	0
Tetracycline	≤ 1-16	≤ 1	≤ 1	6
Sulfamethoxazole	64-512	256	> 512	40
Trimethoprim/sulfamethoxazole	≤ 0.25-4	≤ 0.25	≤ 0.25	1

[a] n.c., no CLSI resistance breakpoints are available for these drugs; the percentage of resistance to penicillin and ampicillin is based on the occurrence of the β-lactam resistance gene blaROB-1.

Table 2. MICs for 11 antimicrobial agents of the *Actinobacillus pleuropneumoniae* clinical strains isolated during 1997–2004 (Gutiérrez-Martín et al., 2006).

Antimicrobial	No. of isolates with MIC of (µg/mL)																MIC_{50}	MIC_{90}	% Resistance
	0.03	0.06	0.12	0.25	0.5	1	2	4	8	16	32	64	128	256	512	> 512			
PEN			< 3	5	27	129	30		2		3	8 >	22				1	64	–
AMOX		<		28	154	10	3		1		3 >	30					0.5	64	–
CEP					< 184	16	15	8	4	│ 1	1 >						0.5	2	0.4
TET				< 1	9	23	6	2	19	│ 48	53	67	1 >				32	64	73.8
STR						< 1			1	38	150	14	1 >	24			32	256	–
GEN		<						55	153 >	│ 21							8	8	9.2
ERY	<		1				7	177 >	44								4	> 4	–
TMP						< 216	1		1			1 >	10				≤ 1	≤ 1	–
NAL						< 1	180	39	1	1 >	7						2	4	–
FIS											< 39	108	39	5	│ 3 >	35	64	> 512	16.6
FFN*			< 85	90	32	22			│				>				0.25	0.5	0

(|): Lines indicate breakpoint for resistance when available; (<): minimum concentration used; (>): maximum concentration used. Abbreviations: PEN, penicillin; AMOX, amoxicillin; CEP, cephalothin; TET, tetracycline; STR, streptomycin; GEN, gentamicin; ERY, erythromycin; TMP, trimethoprim; NAL, nalidixic acid; FIS, sulfisoxazole; FFN, florfenicol.

Table 3. Penetration of antimicrobials in the lung.

Antimicrobial group	**Example**	**Penetration at the site of action**†	**Reference**
Fluoroquinolones	Marbofloxacin/Danofloxacin	+++	Baggot et al., 2000
β-lactam antibiotics	Amoxicillin	++*	
Cephalosporins	Ceftiofur	++*	
Amphenicols	Florfenicol	+++	
Lincosamides	Lincomycin	+++	
"Classic" macrolides	Tilmicosin	+++	
"New" macrolides	Tulathromycin	+++	
Sulphonamides	Sulfadimethoxin	++	
Pleuromutilins	Tiamulin	+++	
Tetracyclines	Doxycycline	+++	
Aminoglycosides	Gentamicin	+	

† Bronchial secretions and pulmonary alveoli.
– no, + low, ++ intermediate and +++ high penetration.
* Higher penetration in inflamed tissues.

Table 4. Probability of clinical success for antimicrobials in the treatment of APP infections.

Antimicrobial group	**Example**	**PK/PD parameter and threshold value**	**Probability of success**
Fluoroquinolones	Marbofloxacin Danofloxacin	Cmax/MIC > 10	+++
Cephalosporins	Ceftiofur	T > MIC (40-50 % of the dose interval)	+++
Phenicols	Florfenicol	T > MIC (40-50 % of the dose interval) and AUC/MIC > 100-125	+++
Lincosamides	Lincomycin	T > MIC (40-50 % of the dose interval)	-
"Classic" macrolides	Tilmicosin	T > MIC (40-50 % of the dose interval)	++/+++
"New" macrolides	Tulathromycin	T > MIC (40-50 % of the dose interval) and AUC/MIC > 100-125	+++
Sulphonamides	Sulfadiazine	T > MIC (40-50 % of the dose interval)	-/+
Sulphonamides + Diaminopyrimidines	Sulfadiazine + Trimethoprim	T > MIC (40-50 % of the dose interval)	+/++
Pleuromutilins	Tiamulin	T > MIC (40-50 % of the dose interval)	+/++
Tetracyclines	Doxycycline	T > MIC (40-50 % of the dose interval)	-/+
Aminoglycosides	Gentamicin	Cmax/MIC > 10	-/+

Probability of success: - failure, + low, ++ intermediate and +++ high.

Table 5. MIC_{50} and MIC_{90} values and range (μg/ml) for antimicrobial drugs against *M. hyopneumoniae* as described by several authors (Burch, 2012).

Antimicrobial	Ref. strain MIC	MIC_{50}	MIC_{90}	Range
Chlortetracycline	12.5 —	12.5 0.39	≥ 100 1.56	0.78- ≥ 100 < 0.024-3.125
Oxytetracycline	0.78 0.25 —	0.78 0.25 0.078	6.25 1 0.31	0.1-12.5 0.025-1 0.039-0.63
Tiamulin	≤ 0.0125 0.025 — — 0.03	≤ 0.0125 0.05 0.039 0.006 ≤ 0.015	0.05 0.05 0.078 0.048 0.12	≤ 0.0125-0.05 0.01-0.1 0.039-0.16 < 0.006-0.097 ≤ 0.015-0.12
Valnemulin	— —	0.0024 < 0.006	0.0049 < 0.006	0.0024-0.0098 < 0.006
Tylosin	≤ 0.0125 0.025 — 0.03	0.025 0.1 0.16 0.06	0.05 0.25 0.31 0.5	≤ 0.0125-0.1 0.025-0.25 0.16-0.63 ≤ 0.015- > 1.0
Tilmicosin	0.1 — 0.25	0.1 0.39 0.25	0.39 1.56 0.5	≤ 0.0125-0.39 < 0.024-3.125 ≤ 0.25- > 16
Tylvalosin	≤ 0.0125	≤ 0.0125	≤ 0.0125	≤ 0.0125-0.05
Josamycin	—	0.048	0.097	< 0.006-0.195
Tulathromycin	—	0.03	0.06	≤ 0.004-0.125
Lincomycin	0.025 — — ≤ 0.06	0.025 0.31 0.048 ≤ 0.06	0.1 0.63 0.097 ≤ 0.06	≤ 0.0125-0.39 0.31-0.63 < 0.006-0.39 ≤ 0.06- > 8.0
Enrofloxacin	0.05 0.03	0.025 0.03	0.05 0.5	0.01-0.1 0.015- > 1.0
Danofloxacin	0.025	0.025	0.05	0.01-0.05

Table 6. MIC breakpoints against certain *Mycoplasma* species as suggested by several investigators (Hannan, 2000).

Mycoplasma species	Antimicrobial agent	Breakpoint (µg/ml)			Investigators
		Sensitive	Intermediate	Resistant	
M. gallisepticum *M. synoviae* *M. iowae* *M. meleagridis*	Oxytetracycline Erythromycin Oleandomycin Roxithromycin Spiramycin Lincomycin Josamycin Tylosin Kitasamycin Enrofloxacin Oxolinic acid	≤ 4–8 ≤ 1–4 ≤ 1–4 ≤ 1–4 ≤ 2–8 ≤ 2–8 ≤ 2–8 ≤ 1 ≤ 8–17 ≤ 1 ≤ 2–4	≤ 8 ≤ 4 ≤ 4 ≤ 4 ≤ 8 ≤ 8 ≤ 8 ≤ 17 ≤ 4	> 8 > 4 > 4 > 4 > 8 > 8 > 8 > 1 > 17 > 1 > 4	Kempf et al., 1989
M. hyorhinis	Tetracycline Chloramphenicol Erythromycin	≤ 1 ≤ 4 ≤ 1	≤ 4 ≤ 8 ≤ 2	≥ 32 ≥ 16 ≥ 4	Ter Laak et al., 1991
M. hyopneumoniae *M. flocculare*	Clindamycin Ofloxacin Ciprofloxacin	≤ 1 ≤ 1 ≤ 1	≤ 2 ≤ 4 ≤ 2	≥ 8 ≥ 16 ≥ 16	
M. bovis *M. dispar* *U. diversum*	Tetracycline Chloramphenicol Streptomycin	≤ 1 ≤ 4 ≤ 4	2–4 8 8–16	≥ 8 ≥ 16 ≥ 32	Ter Laak et al., 1993
M. gallisepticum *M. synoviae*	Enrofloxacin	≤ 0.5 ≤ 4	≤ 1 8	≥ 2 ≥ 16	
M. iowae *M. bovis* *M. agalactiae* *M. hyorhinis* *M. hyopneumoniae* *M. hyosynoviae*	Oxytetracycline Flumequine Tylosin Tiamulin	≤ 4 ≤ 4 ≤ 1 ≤ 8	8 8 ≤ 2 –	≥ 16 ≥ 16 ≥ 4 ≥ 16	Hannan et al., 1997

The breakpoint cited for each antibiotic applies to all the *Mycoplasma* species tested by each investigator.

Table 7. MIC of *Pasteurella Multocida* of 132 isolates recovered from lungs of pigs with pneumonia in Spain from 2003 to 2004 (Lizarazo et al., 2006).

Antimicrobial	0.12	0.25	0.5	1	2	4	8	16	32	64	128	256	512	MIC_{50}	MIC_{90}	% Resistance
PEN	< 91	33	1	1	1	—	—	1 >	4	—	—	—	—	≤ 0.12	0.25	3.8
AMP	—	< 119	6	1	—	1	—	1 >	1	4	—	—	—	≤ 0.25	≤ 0.25	3.0
XNL	—	—		< 131	1	—	>	—	—	—	—	—	—	≤ 0.5	≤ 0.5	0
GEN	—	—	—	< 7	85	29	11 >	—	—	—	—	—	—	2	4	0
APR	—	—	—	—	—	< 1	11	76	34 >	10	—	—	—	16	32	ND
NEO	—	—	—	—	—	< 56	55	21	>	—	—	—		8	16	0
SPE	—	—	—	—	—	—	< 21	84	18	2 >	1	7	—	16	16	5.3
CTET	—	—	< 12	33	46	24	16 >	1	1	—	—	—	—	2	8	0.7
OXY	—	<	8	21	56	15	13 >	19	—	—	—	—	—	2	> 8	14.4
CLI	—	<	—	—	>	132	—	—	—	—	—	—	—	> 2	> 2	ND
TYLT*	—	—	—	—	—	—	—							10	20	ND
ERY	—	<	—	9	81	37	5 >	—	—	—	—	—	—	2	4	3.8
TYL	—	—	—	—	—	< 114	12	6	>	—	—	—	-	≤ 4	8	0
ENRO	< 132	-	-	>	-	-	-	-	-	-				≤ 0.12	≤ 0.12	0
SCP	-	-	-	-	-	-	-	-	< 2	7	22	9 >	92	> 256	> 256	69.7
SDM	-	-	-	-	-	-	-	-	< 6	11	5	2 >	108	> 256	> 256	81.8
STZ	-	-	-	-	-	-	-	-	> 9	8	4	5 >	106	> 256	> 256	80.3
FFC	-	< 26	92	14	-	-	>	-	-	-	-	-	-	0.5	1	0
TIA	-	-	-	-	-	< 2	18	46	61 >	5	-	-	-	16	32	50.0

Numbers to the right of the vertical line (breakpoint line) for a particular antimicrobial indicate that this was the highest concentration tested for which *Pasteurella multocida* was detected.

PEN = Penicillin. AMP = Ampicillin. XNL = Ceftiofur. GEN = Gentamicin. APR = Apramycin. NEO = Neomycin. SPE = Spectinomycin. CTET = Chlortetracycline. OXY = Oxytetracycline. CLI = Clindamycin. TYLT = Tylosin tartrate. ERY = Erythromycin. TYL = Tilmicosin. ENRO = Enrofloxacin. SCP = Sulfachlorpiridazine. SDM = Sulfadimethoxine. STZ = Sultathiazole. COT = Trimethoprim-sulfamethoxazole. FFC = Florfenicol. TIA = Tiamulin:

< = Minimum concentration tested.
> = Maximum concentration tested.

* For TYLT, only the MIC_{50} and MIC_{90} value are shown, because the dilution range of this antimicrobial agent was different from that of the remaining compounds.

ND = Not determined as there is no breakpoint for this antimicrobial and this bacterial species.

Table 8. Probability of clinical success for antimicrobials in the treatment of MH and PM infections.

Antimicrobial group	Example	PK/PD parameter and threshold value	Probability of success for MH	Probability of success for PM
Fluoroquinolones	Marbofloxacin / Danofloxacin	Cmax/MIC > 10	++/+++	+++
Cephalosporins	Ceftiofur	T > MIC (40-50 % of the dose interval)	–	+++
Phenicols	Florfenicol	T > MIC (40-50 % of the dose interval) and AUC/MIC > 100-125	+/++	+++
"Classic" macrolides	Tilmicosin	T > MIC (40-50 % of the dose interval)	+++	+/++
"New" macrolides	Tulathromycin	T > MIC (40-50 % of the dose interval) and AUC/MIC > 100-125	+++	+++
Lincosamides	Lincomycin	T > MIC (40-50 % of the dose interval)	+++	–
Sulphonamides	Sulfadiazine	T > MIC (40-50 % of the dose interval)	+	–/+
Sulphonamides + Diaminopyrimidines	Sulfadiazine + Trimethoprim	T > MIC (40-50 % of the dose interval)	++	+/++
Pleuromutilins	Tiamulin	T > MIC (40-50 % of the dose interval)	++	–/+
Tetracyclines	Doxycicline	T > MIC (40-50 % of the dose interval)	+/++	++/+++
Aminoglycosides	Gentamicin	Cmax/MIC > 10	-	+/++*

* Not usually applied due to the potential toxicity problem after parenteral administration.

Tabla 9. Comparison between several antibiotics used for prevention and treatment of enzootic pneumonia. The key paremeter is the reduction in lung lesions (%).

Antimicrobial	Reference	Dose (mg/kg p.v./day)	Inclusion rate in feed ration (ppm)	Prevention Lesion reduction (%)	Treatment Lesion reduction (%)	Detection
Chlortetracycline (CTC)	Thacker et al., 2000	22	550	95	36	—
Tiamulin	Schuller et al., 1977	5	100	35	—	—
Tiamulin	Simon et al., 1990	10	200	58	—	—
Tiamulin	Simon et al., 1990	10	200	—	57-92	Yes
Tiamulin	Hannan et al., 1982	20 (g)	400 (e)	—	98	Yes
Tiamulin + CTC	Miller & Stipkovits 1990	5 + 15	100 + 300	97	—	Yes
Tiamulin + CTC	Stipkovits et al., 2001	5 + 20	100 + 400	—	76	Yes
Tylosin	Hannan et al., 1982	100 (g)	2000 (e)	—	95	Yes

Tabla 9. Comparative of several antibiotics used for prevention and treatment of enzootic pneumonia. The key paremeter is the reduction of the pulmonary lesion (%). Continuation.

Antimicrobial	**Reference**	**Dose (mg/kg p.v./day)**	**Inclusion rate in feed ration (ppm)**	**Prevention Lesion reduction (%)**	**Treatment Lesion reduction (%)**	**Detection**
Tylosin + sulphadimine	Miller & Stipkovits, 1990	5 + 15	100 + 300	52	—	Yes
Lyncomicine	Kubo et al., 1990	4,4	88	26	—	—
		8,8	176	41	—	—
Lyncomicine + CTC	Stipkovits et al., 2001	5	100	—	24	Yes
		20	400	—	—	—
Valnemuline	Morgan et al., 1996	10	200	45	—	—
		15	300	43	—	—
		20	400	71	—	—
	Burrows et al., 2001	10	200	79	—	—
		10	200	—	38	—
Valnemuline + CTC	Stipkovits et al., 2001	3,25 +	75	—	90	Yes
		20	400	—	—	—
Acetylisovaleryltylosin	Burrows et al., 2002	2,5	50	45	51	—
		5	100	—	32	—
Tilmicosin	Stipkovits et al., 2001	15	300	—	60	Yes
		20	400	—	60	Yes

(e): estimated.

(g): tube administration.

3 Treatment of digestive diseases

Treatment of digestive diseases

3

General concepts

Digestive tract

The treatment of gastrointestinal disorders focuses on locating the disease in a segment of the digestive tract and determining its cause. A specific therapeutic plan can then be designed to solve each clinical case. Describing all the diseases that can affect the digestive system is out of the scope of this book. This chapter will only address the diseases in which microorganisms are decisive in their pathogenesis. In this case, antibiotics can be indicated in the treatment and it will be necessary to design the most appropriate dosage regimen to address each specific clinical case (Merck, 1991).

Gastrointestinal diseases due to microorganisms generally cause diarrhoea through various mechanisms that need to be known in order to understand, diagnose and treat them. The physiopathological mechanisms that cause scouring are an increase in permeability, hypersecretion and osmosis. Hypermotility is often a secondary phenomenon.

INCREASE IN PERMEABILITY

In healthy animals there is a continuous flow of water and electrolytes through the intestinal mucosa. Both the secretory flow (movement from the blood to the intestines) and absorption (movement from the intestines to the blood) occur simultaneously. In a clinically normal animal, the flows of absorption exceed those of secretion, giving rise to net absorption. The inflammation of the intestine can be accompanied with an increase in the "size of the pores" in the mucosa, thus allowing an increase of the flow through the membrane ("escape") across the pressure gradient from the blood to the intestinal lumen. If the secreted amount exceeds the capacity of absorption of the intestines, diarrhoea occurs. The size of the material that escapes through the mucosa varies, depending on the magnitude of the increase in its size. Considerable increases in the size of the pores will allow plasma proteins to be released, resulting in enteropathies with a loss of proteins (e.g. bovine paratuberculosis) (Blood and Radostits, 1992).

HYPERSECRETION

Hypersecretion is defined as an increase in the intestinal flow of liquids and electrolytes from the blood to the intestines, which occurs regardless of the changes in permeability, capacity of absorption or osmotic gradients that are generated exogenously. Enterotoxic colibacillosis is an example of a diarrhoeic disease that results in intestinal hypersecretion. These bacteria produce enterotoxins that stimulate the intestinal epithelium to secrete more fluids than those that can be absorbed in the intestine. In this case, the epithelium remains intact, along with its digestion and absorption abilities. The fluid that is secreted is alkaline, isotonic and free from inflammatory exudates. The fact that the epithelium is intact is beneficial to the animal, since the oral administration of a liquid that contains glucose, amino-acids and sodium will cause absorption even in the presence of hypersecretion (Fairbrother, 2005).

OSMOTIC DIARRHOEA

Osmotic diarrhoea takes place when an inadequate absorption gives rise to an accumulation of solutes in the intestinal lumen, which causes water retention due to its osmotic activity. It is observed in any disorder that gives rise to a deficient absorption or digestion of nutrients. Deficient absorption is the failure of digestion and absorption, due to a lesion of the enterocytes. Several epitheliotropic viruses, such as coronaviruses or rotaviruses, infect and destroy the enterocytes. The different types of viruses are able to infect enterocytes at different stages of maturation (from the crypts to the tip of the villi). The regeneration of the epithelium will require more time after an infection by parvovirus (it affects enterocytes from the crypt to the tip) than in an infection by a virus that only affects mature enterocytes at the tip of the intestinal villi (coronavirus and rotavirus). A deficient intestinal absorption can also be the cause of a defect in the capacity of absorption, such as diffuse inflammatory disorders (e.g. eosinophilic enteritis) or neoplastic conditions (lymphosarcoma).

The infectious diseases that affect the small intestine in species of veterinary interest are very important as they have high economic costs due to their high prevalence. These costs are derived from the increase in mortality and the negative impact on the production parameters in production animals (Constable, 2004).

The administration of intravenous fluids and rehydrating solutions by oral route are essential therapeutic measures in the treatment of many of these diseases. However, the administration of antibiotics to treat infectious diseases that affect the intestine (especially the small intestine) could be controversial (Constable, 2004). In this book about antibiotic therapy, several clinical cases of digestive diseases that affect both the small and the large intestine in pigs will be described. Indeed, there are three major regions of clinical significance; the upper and mid small intestine (duodenum and jejunum) for *Escherichia coli* (EC) infections, the lower small intestine (ileum) for *Lawsonia intracellularis* (LI) infections and the large intestine (colon) for *Brachyspira hyodysenteriae* (BH) and *Brachyspira pilosicoli* (BP) infections. In addition, the most appropriate antimicrobial therapy depending on the therapeutic objective to be achieved will be discussed. The therapeutic objective may vary from prevention to treatment of the disease in the affected animals and even the eradication of the disease.

Penetration of the antibiotic at the site of action

In the introductory chapter, we have seen that pharmacokinetics enables us to predict the blood or plasma concentration of a drug after its administration, but it does not allow us to know the concentrations in the other tissues of the organism at the same kinetic times, unless tissue samples are also taken. When dealing with the treatment of an infection in the digestive tract, it is indispensable to know where the pathogen is located exactly (small or large intestine) and which concentrations are reached in each segment of the intestine. There are very limited data available on antibiotic concentrations reached in the intestines. There is, however, more information on concentrations in faecal or colonic contents, as these data are now required for regulatory purposes, for environmental risk assessments, the establishment of microbiological maximum residue limits and more recently for PK/PD integration regarding efficacy. The antibiotic concentration that can be reached depending on the route of administration (oral versus parenteral) in the target tissues will be reviewed.

ADMINISTRATION BY PARENTERAL ROUTE

Any antibiotic administered by parenteral route can reach the intestinal tract by two routes. The first one is by biliary route, either as an active substance or as a metabolite (active or not) after hepatic biotransformation. As an example, ceftiofur reaches the jejunum by this route and the concentration observed in this part of the small intestine is 9-12 % of the concentration observed in plasma at the same kinetic time (Schionning, 1994). The second route through which an antibiotic can reach the intestine is by being actively secreted into the intestinal tract by the epithelial cells of the mucosa (Martínez-Jiménez, 2006), as occurs in the case of quinolones. Thus, the concentration of danofloxacin after its parenteral administration is higher in the gastrointestinal contents of pigs than in the plasma at the same kinetic times. Figures 1, 2, 3 and 4 show the pharmacokinetics of danofloxacin after its intravenous administration as well as its concentration in various intestinal segments in pigs (Lindecrona, 2000) after an experimental infection by *Salmonella thyphimuirum*. The first element that can be highlighted is that the pharmacokinetics is different in healthy and sick pigs. Sick animals eliminate the drug more slowly than healthy animals and the concentration of drug in the mucosa and intestinal contents of healthy and infected pigs is higher than the plasma concentration at the same kinetic times.

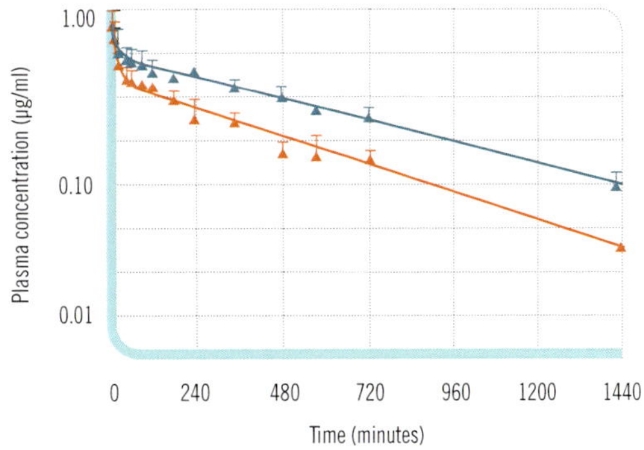

Figure 1. Plasma level curves in healthy pigs (red triangles) and in pigs infected with *Salmonella thyphimurium* (green triangles) observed after the intravenous administration of a dose of 2.40 mg/kg live weight/day of danofloxacin. The represent values the mean of 3 animals.

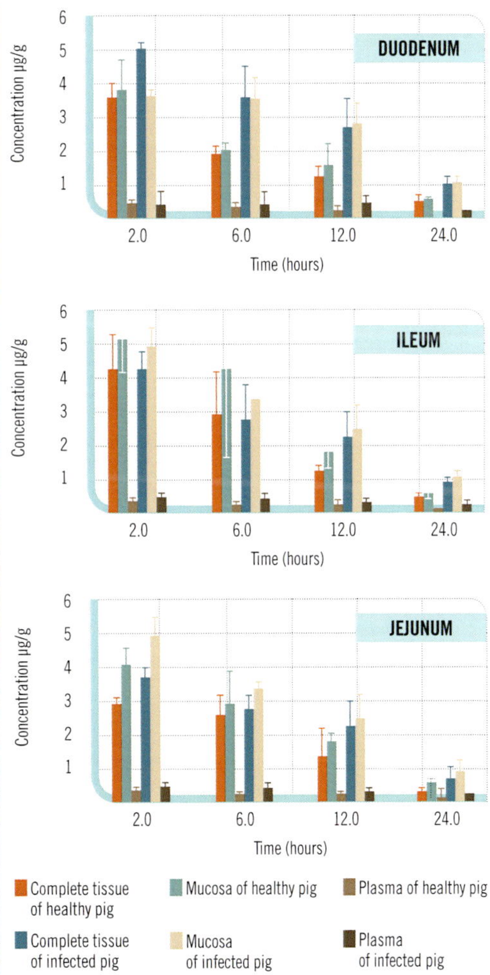

Figure 2. Mean danofloxacin concentration in plasma (µg/ml), complete tissue and mucosa of the duodenum, ileum and jejunum (µg/g) in healthy pigs and pigs infected with *Salmonella thyphimurium*, observed after the administration of a dose of 2.40 mg/kg b.w. of danofloxacin by intravenous route. The values represent the mean of 3 animals.

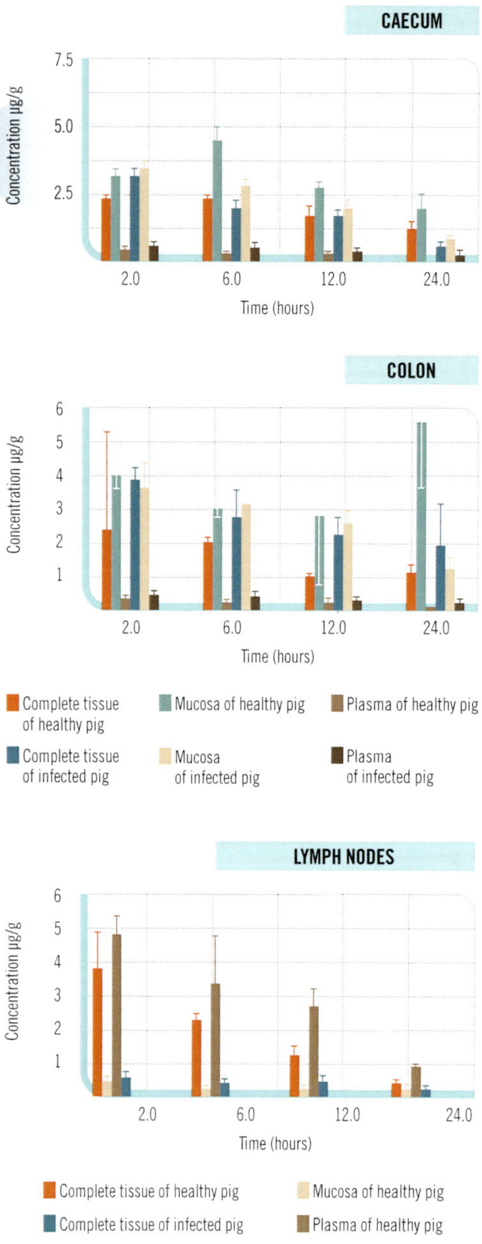

Figure 3. Mean danofloxacin concentration in plasma (μg/ml), complete tissue and mucosa of the caecum and colon (μg/g) as well as in the lymph nodes of healthy pigs and pigs infected with *Salmonella thyphimurium*, observed after the administration of a dose of 2.40 mg/kg b.w. of danofloxacin by intravenous route. The values represent the mean of 3 animals.

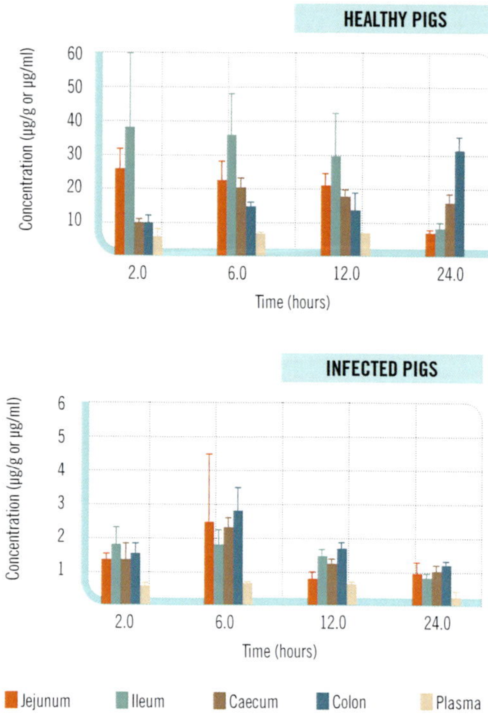

Figure 4. Mean danofloxacin concentration in plasma (μg/ml) and in the contents of the ileum, jejunum, caecum and colon (μg/ml) of healthy pigs and pigs infected with *Salmonella thyphimurium*, observed after the administration of a dose of 2.40 mg/kg b.w. of danofloxacin by intravenous route. The values represent the mean of 3 animals.

ADMINISTRATION BY ORAL ROUTE

In general, the antibiotics that are administered orally in feed concentrate after going through the intestine. Thus, an antibiotic administered at a dose of 100 ppm in feed, which is not absorbed and does not undergo a metabolisation process in the intestine (e.g. destruction by intestinal enzymes) shows a concentration in faeces of 250 ppm (Burch, 2003). However, the concentration in each part of the gastrointestinal tract (expressed as μg/ml of intestinal content) is very variable and will perfectly reflect the physiological processes (absorption of water, excretion, etc.) that take place in each intestinal segment (Fig. 5).

Figure 6 shows the concentration of penicillin in the gastrointestinal tract of pigs after administering a single oral dose of 15.9 mg/kg of procaine penicillin suspension to pigs of 60-80 kg body weight (McKellar, 1987) previously fasted for 12 hours. High quantities of the penicillin in suspension entered the duodenum, jejunum and ileum at 15, 30 and 120 minutes, respectively, after its administration. This concentration decreased quickly in the duodenum and jejunum after reaching the maximum value and this drug was under the limit for detection after 60 and 120 minutes in the duodenum and jejunum, respectively. However, a comparatively steady concentration was achieved in the ileum. On the other hand, penicillin concentration in the colon was very low (< 0.7 µg/ml), probably due to the absorption and breakdown of the drug in the gastrointestinal tract.

It is possible to observe an effect of dilution in the stomach and small intestine as well as a progressive increase in the concentration as we approach the most distal parts of the intestine, unless a breakdown of the active substance takes place due to the acid environment, enzymes, bacteria and binding. In addition to the actual concentration of antibiotic, it is also necessary to take into account how long the drug is present in each intestinal segment. This parameter will depend on the time of transit in each part of the digestive tract. Gastric emptying time can be slowed by age (Snoeck, 2004), feeding (Casteel, 1998) and formulation (Davis, 2001). It is accepted in the literature that liquids pass through the gut more quickly than micro-pellets. Davis (2001) reported a transit time of 3–4 hours for liquids and Snoeck (2004) reported more than 7 hours for micro-pellets in meal. This observation is relevant taking into account the physiological changes that take place in a pig during the first four weeks of life. Suckling pigs have a faster gastric emptying time than weaned pigs. However, the gastric emptying time is similar in adults and young pigs from three weeks after weaning (Snoeck, 2004). The drug is present in the small intestine

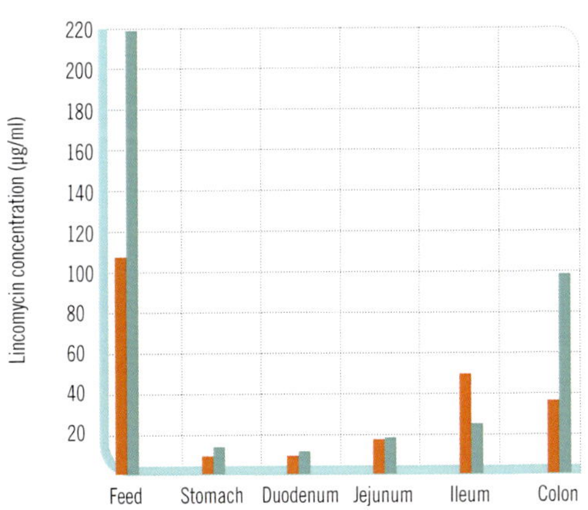

Figure 5. Mean lincomycin concentration in the contents of the stomach, duodenum, ileum, jejunum and colon (µg/ml), observed after the oral administration of lincomycin mixed with feed at a dose of 100 ppm (orange bars) and 200 ppm (green bars).

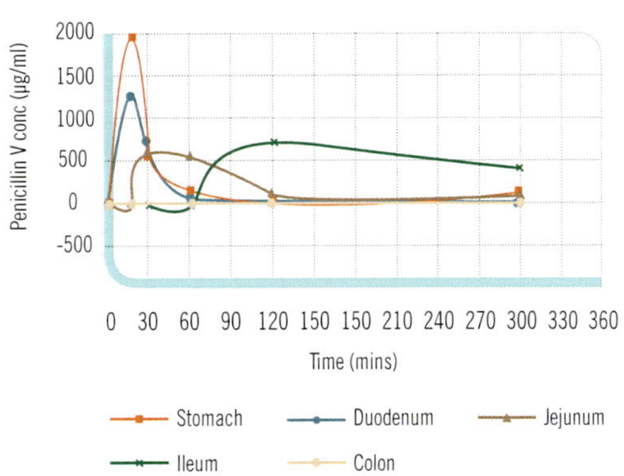

Figure 6. Concentrations of penicillin (µg/ml) in the gastrointestinal tract of pigs following the administration of a single oral dose of procaine penicilin suspension at 15.9 mg/kg b.w. (McKellar et al., 1987).

for 12 hours after eating the medicated feed. Intestinal transit is much slower in the colon (24-48 hours) and, as explained previously, drugs tend to concentrate due to the absorption of liquids that takes place in this segment. In addition, there are a great number of bacteria that can destroy drugs in the colon and the binding of some antibiotics to faeces can reduce their availability when they should exert their pharmacological effect (Del Castillo, 1998; Burch, 2003).

Treatment of acute diseases affecting the small intestine

Description of the clinical picture

HISTORY

- Piglets in a nursery unit coming from one sow origin. The capacity of the unit is 8000 places distributed in rooms of 1000 piglets. Seven rooms have animals allocated in them and one is empty and ready to allocate animals
- Age of the affected animals: between 5 and 6 weeks.
- Percentage of dead pigs until the detection of the problem in the batches of 5 and 6 weeks of age: 1 %.

CLINICAL SIGNS OBSERVED

- Overall, dehydrated animals or animals that look sick can be found in the batches of animals that are between 5 and 6 weeks of age (Fig. 7).
- The affected animals do not have fever but their general state is deteriorating rapidly.
- The caretaker found 5 and 8 dead pigs the day we are notified of the problem.
- 20 animals show the same clinical signs in the batches previously described.
- A necropsy of the animals is performed and the following can be observed::
    - Small intestine filled with liquid.
    - The carcasses are extremely dehydrated (sunken eyes).
    - The mesenteric lymph nodes are congestive ("black").

Presumptive diagnosis

- Enteritis caused probably by gram-negative bacteria (*Salmonella* spp. and/or *Escherichia coli*) and/or a virus (rotavirus or coronavirus) and/or parasites (*Cryptosporidium* and coccidia). The bacteria that are most likely involved in this clinical case are *Escherichia coli* (EC). The clinical incidence of digestive problems due to these bacteria is maximum at this range age (Fig. 8).

BRIEF DESCRIPTION OF POSTWEANING ENTERIC COLIBACILLOSIS IN PIGS

Postweaning diarrhoea (PWD) caused by *Escherichia coli* (EC), also called postweaning enteric colibacillosis, is an important cause of death in weaned pigs and occurs worldwide. EC infection in weaned piglets may also manifest as non-severe diarrhoea, which usually occurs during the first week of the postweaning period and often results in decreased weight gain. Several factors such as the stress of weaning, the lack of antibodies originating from the sow's milk and dietary changes contribute to the severity of this disease. Recently, an increase in the incidence of outbreaks of severe diarrhoea caused by EC has been observed worldwide. Other factors contributing to the increased number of outbreaks of this more severe form of diarrhoea are not yet fully understood. These may include a more

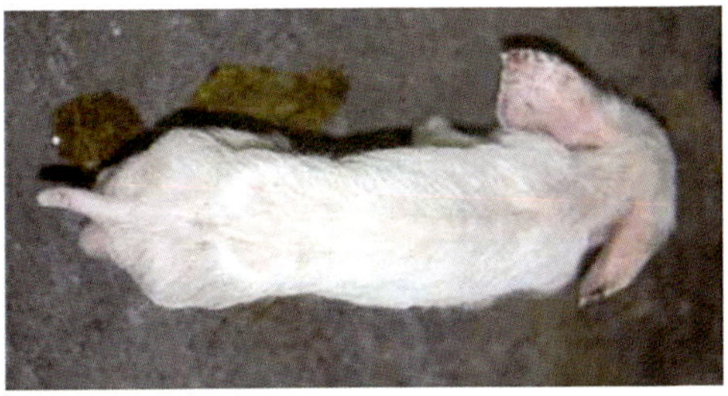

Figure 7. Dehydrated animal that can be found in the batches of animals that are between 5 and 6 weeks of age.

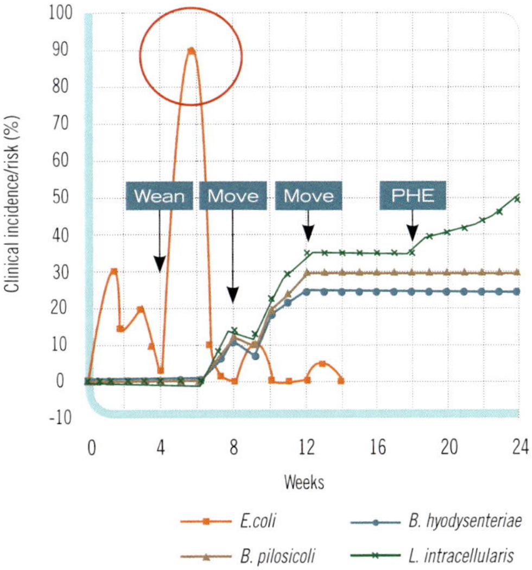

Figure 8. Epidemiology of bacterial digestive disease in pigs (Aarestup et al., 2008).

effective EC colonisation of the intestine due to the changes in feed regimens following weaning. For instance, on farms where husbandry measures such as addition of higher levels of protein of animal source, plasma, acidifying agents, and zinc oxide are used at weaning, peaks of diarrhoea and enteric colibacillosis complicated by shock may be delayed until 3 weeks after weaning, and even 6–8 weeks after weaning, at the time when the pigs enter the growing barns (Fairbrother, unpublished results).

The presence of enterotoxigenic EC (ETEC) in the environment of pigs is an important factor in the development of diarrhoea since these bacteria are able to survive for at least 6 months in the environment if they are protected by manure (Van Beers-Schreurs, 1992). Moreover, ETEC may be disseminated by the feed, other pigs, or other animal species (Bertschinger, 1999). For this reason, when designing preventive measures at farm level to cope with this disease, strict biosecurity measures should be established to decrease the bacterial load in the facilities before newly weaned piglets are transferred to the unit. In addition, diet is one of the most important factors influencing the course of the disease in these animals. "Protective factors" have been described in the literature, such as a diet rich in milk products and energy (Tzipori, 1980), dried plasma added to the feed (Van Beers-Schreurs, 1992) and the presence of organic acidifiers (Giesting and Easter, 1985). In contrast, the presence of other ingredients in the feed, such as soybeans, seems to be a risk factor for the occurrence of PWD. The addition of zinc oxide at levels above 2400 ppm in the feed decreases the severity of PWD although zinc sulphate and organic zinc are potentially toxic (Holm and Poulsen, 1996).

Finally, there may also be bacterial factors that contribute to the recent upsurge in outbreaks of severe disease such as changes in the characteristics of the EC isolates associated with PWD and the possible emergence of more virulent clones. Regardless of the cause of this upsurge, it will be primordial to develop alternative prophylactic strategies for an effective control of this disease in pigs. As previously commented, these strategies must focus on biosecurity measures, reviewing the diet fed to the animals and the rational use of antibiotics to control this clinical problem.

Initial treatment

SYMPTOMATIC

- Administration of saline solution by intraperitoneal route, adjusting the amount administered to the hydration status. The subcutaneous route was also used in animals with mild dehydration.

AETIOLOGIC

- Administration of and antibiotic according to the manufacturer's specifications. The parenteral and oral routes can be used in the most and least affected animals, respectively. This point will be discussed in depth further on.

CRITICAL REVIEW OF THE TREATMENT AND THERAPY OPTIMISATION

Symptomatic treatment

In general, diarrhoea occurs in the small intestine with a considerable loss of fluids that leads to dehydration of the animals. Dehydration can be the final cause of death in affected animals and rehydration is therefore essential. In this case, saline solution was used. It is a reasonable option but it would have been better to use lactated Ringer's solution to compensate the metabolic acidosis that the animals probably present. On some occasions, the use of a rehydrating solution by oral route may also be indicated. Thus, after solving the acute case, it would have been best to continue oral rehydration for a few more days.

Aetiological treatment

The aetiological treatment must aim at blocking the main aetiopathogenic mechanism in each clinical case. In this case:

1. If diarrhoea is caused by a virus (rotavirus and/or coronavirus), there are no antiviral drugs that can block its multiplication. Therefore, the treatment can only be symptomatic (rehydration), given that these viral infections are self-limited (they last for less than a week) since the enterocytes (coming from the crypts) that substitute the infected ones are resistant to the infection by the virus (they have high levels of interferon alpha).
2. If diarrhoea is caused by *Cryptosporidium*, there is no aetiological treatment available in swine (although halofuginone lactate is authorised in calves), but it is necessary to administer the symptomatic treatment previously described.
3. If diarrhoea is caused by gram-negative bacteria, it seems reasonable to think that an antibiotic treatment is indicated either by oral or by parenteral route. This point will be discussed in depth next.

CRITICAL REVIEW OF THE ADMINISTRATION OF ANTIBIOTICS IN THE TREATMENT

NEED TO USE ANTIBIOTICS

As previously explained, the aetiology of diarrhoea in young pigs can be caused by bacteria, viruses and/or parasites. Mixed infections with enteric pathogens are therefore often diagnosed in pigs suffering from diarrhoea (Blood and Radostits, 1992; Constable, 2004).

It has been observed that calves suffering from diarrhoea show an abnormal overgrowth of coliform bacteria in the small intestine, regardless of their age or of the exact cause of the diarrhoea. More precisely, the amount of *Escherichia coli* increases by 5 to 10,000 times in the duodenum, jejunum and ileum of the calves presenting with clinical signs of neonatal diarrhoea, even if the diarrhoea was not initially caused by enterotoxigenic strains of *Escherichia* coli (Constable, 2004). In addition, the amount of coliform bacteria in the study did not change in the large intestine and it can be assumed that a similar situation is observed in young pigs. This situation may be even worse when the primary aetiological agent is *Escherichia coli*. Thus, the antibiotic must be able to decrease the bacterial load in the gastrointestinal tract to improve the clinical outcome.

The administration of antibiotics in young pigs affected by diarrhoea is indicated in order to control the growth of coliform bacteria, regardless of the primary aetiological agent (viruses, other bacteria and/or parasites) that has triggered the signs of diarrhoea. If the primary aetiological agent involved is *Salmonella* spp., it would be advisable to choose an antimicrobial agent that is effective to control both microorganisms. In conclusion, there is a generalised consensus in the literature on the need to use antibiotics when designing a therapy in clinical cases of swine colibacillosis (Prescott, 2000). Fortunately, there are many antibiotics available that have shown to be effective for the treatment of this disease. It is possible to use antibiotics that belong to the class of quinolones (enrofloxacin, marbofloxacin and danofloxacin), β-lactam antibiotics (amoxicillin), cephalosporins (ceftiofur and cefquinome), aminoglycosides (neomycin and apramycin), aminocyclitols (spectinomycin), polymyxins (colistin sulphate) and sulphonamides, usually combined with trimethoprim (sulfadiazine + trimethoprim).

Therapeutic approach

The elements that should be taken into consideration are the following:

- The infection is located mainly in the small intestine.
- The selected dosage regimen must have a fast action since the clinical case evolves very quickly. In addition, the treatment must be as short as possible to decrease the probability of generating dysbiosis.

After these considerations, an antibiotic should be chosen to treat this disease. It should have the following characteristics:

- Active against gram-negative microorganisms (mainly *Escherichia coli* and *Salmonella* spp.).
- It must reach sufficient concentrations to have an effect on the small intestine regardless of the administration route (oral or parenteral).

The first question that should be answered is to what animals the antibiotic should be administered. Obviously, these drugs should be administered to all the animals with clinical signs compatible with this disease. In addition, given the short period of incubation of this disease as well as the high mortality in the affected animals, antibiotics should be administered to all the animals in the pens where mortality has been observed. From a strictly pharmacological point of view, it may seem that this is not justified; however, it must be done given the epidemiology and the morbidity/mortality of this disease. This therapeutic approach is metaphylactic and it is highly recommended in the event of an outbreak of swine colibacillosis.

An antibiotic should be chosen taking into account these considerations. In this case, the first characteristic to consider is that the antimicrobial must be active against *Escherichia coli*.

As explained in the first chapter, antimicrobial susceptibility against EC is usually measured with the MIC value. The MIC values of a list of antimicrobials that may be used in an EC outbreak are listed in Table 1.

The second element that needs to be known is the concentration of the antimicrobial that will be reached at the site of action. In this case, the site of action is the intestine and more precisely, the intestinal contents. The penetration of the candidate antimicrobials to treat an EC outbreak at this site after parenteral administration is given in Table 2. Obviously, penetration after oral administration is high for antimicrobials with a low or no absorption (aminoglycosides, polymyxins and aminocyclitols).

The PK/PD parameters of the antimicrobials that may be used should be calculated for each clinical case in order to predict clinical efficacy in a case by case situation. As an example, the different PK/PD parameters calculated for a concentration-dependent antibiotic (danofloxacin) are given next.

PK/PD PARAMETER FOR A CONCENTRATION-DEPENDENT ANTIBIOTIC

A concentration-dependent antibiotic is an antibiotic with an effect on microorganisms that depends on its concentration. In this case, the Cmax/MIC and AUC/MIC ratios are the PK/PD parameters that best correlate with clinical efficacy. In spite of the existing limitations, an AUC/MIC ratio value of 100 is taken as a reference in this case, since there is no precise information available in the literature about the PK/PD parameter values in the treatment of enteric diseases in veterinary medicine (Guyonnet, 2003; Apley, 2005). The value for this parameter is 3.4 (0.43/0.125) for danofloxacin and EC when it is calculated taking into account the maximum plasma concentration. This value is under the threshold value (Cmax/MIC = 10) usually accepted for quinolones. However, danofloxacin concentrates in different parts of the intestine (Figs. 2, 3 and 4). Thus, considering the danofloxacin maximum concentration observed in the mucosa (4.87 µg/ml) and taking into account a Cmax/MIC ratio value of 10 as an indicator of efficacy, the treatment of clinical cases of swine colibacillosis with danofloxacin can be expected to be effective (Cmax /MIC = 39). The two AUC values should also be taken into consideration: on the one hand, the AUCic value (24 hours), which will be calculated as the mean concentration in the small intestine (in the intestinal contents or ic) multiplied by 24 hours, assuming that the infection is located in the intestinal lumen; and on the other hand, the AUCm value (24 hours). This value will be calculated as the mean concentration in the mucosa of the small intestine multiplied by 24 hours. This parameter is also relevant because the microorganism could go through the mucosa (m) and pass to the systemic circulation in case of septicaemic EC. The MIC_{90} value (0.125 µg/ml) will be used in the next calculations (Table 3).

Given the results obtained and considering an AUC/MIC ratio value of 100 as an indicator of efficacy, the treatment can be expected to be effective. These results have been corroborated by clinical trials in which the efficacy of the treatment of this disease with danofloxacin has been unequivocally confirmed. Finally, it is worth mentioning that the concentration of danofloxacin in the intestinal lumen is much higher in healthy pigs than in infected pigs (Fig. 4). In this specific case, this information is not relevant to predict the efficacy of the treatment. However, all the pharmacokinetic studies should be carried out in sick animals because it may not be possible to directly extrapolate the results obtained in healthy animals (pharmacokinetics and distribution to tissues) to every pathological situation, as it is the case here. Indeed, while the studies carried out for an antibiotic in healthy animals may suggest that the treatment can be effective; the clinical trials (conducted in sick animals) may indicate that it is not. This information can help us to explain the possible contradictions that there may be between PK/PD studies (nearly always in healthy animals) and clinical trials (in sick animals) for some antimicrobials.

The probability of clinical success with the antimicrobials that may be used for the treatment of EC infections can be calculated taking into account the pharmacokinetic and pharmacodynamic information provided by the pharmaceutical companies or available in the public domain (Table 4).

The information provided in Table 4 is for guidance only, as each strain has its own MIC value for each antimicrobial. The PK/PD parameters of the antimicrobials that may be used should therefore be calculated for each clinical case and the result should be taken into account to optimise the therapy and choose the best antimicrobial option (see Fig. 14 in chapter 2). In addition, in order to choose an appropriate antimicrobial agent, swine practitioners should know the efficacy of the molecule (previously analysed), the current regulations on the use of antimicrobials in their country and the history of the herd.

Finally, the only factor that is usually taken into consideration to assess the efficacy of a treatment for digestive diseases is the improvement of clinical signs (in general, diarrhoea). However, a very important factor in the treatment of digestive diseases is the reduction in the excretion of pathogens during and after the treatment. This factor is very important since it can reduce the incidence of recurrences. As can be observed in Figure 9, the clinical response (reduction of mortality) is comparable when very different doses of antibiotic are used. However, the excretion of the microorganisms decreases as the dose increases. This point can be taken into account if the summary of product characteristics provides a wide range of doses. It may be more interesting to use higher doses if these lead to a reduced excretion of the pathogen, even if clinical efficacy is the same. This consideration can be very important when the treatment is applied to large populations of pigs that are housed on operations with high densities of animals.

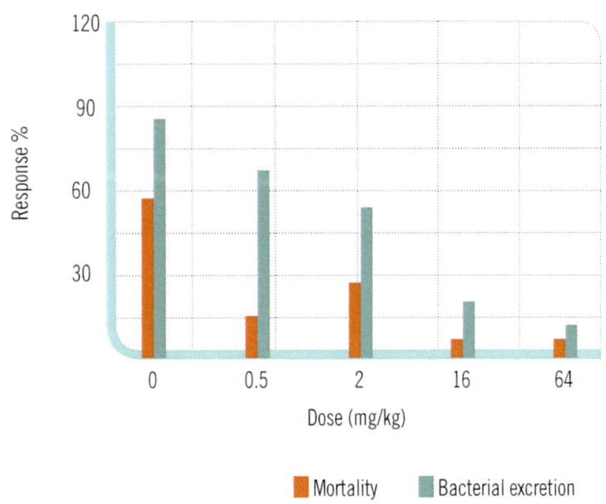

Figure 9. Clinical efficacy (measured as the improvement in the mortality rate) and excretion of *Escherichia coli* (measured as the percentage of pigs excreting the bacteria) observed in pigs after the administration ceftiofur at increasing doses (from 0 to 64 mg/kg) in a model of experimental infection (Yancey, 1990).

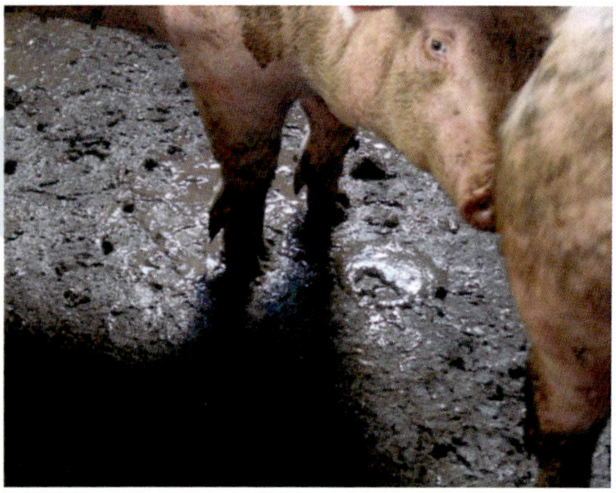

Figure 10

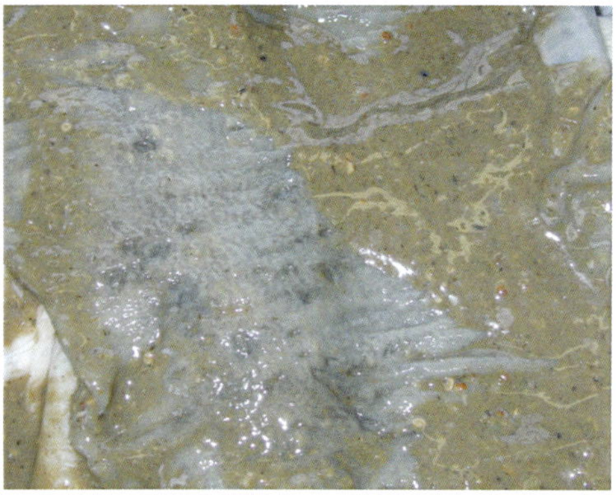

Figure 11

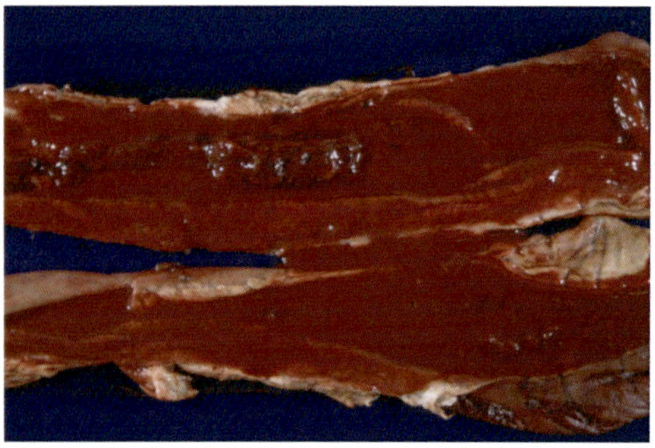

Figure 12

Treatment of chronic diseases affecting the distal part of the small intestine and the large intestine

Description of the clinical picture

HISTORY

- The affected animals were housed in a fattening unit on a farrow-to-finish farm. The farm was free from the Aujeszky's disease virus and was positive to the porcine reproductive and respiratory syndrome virus.
- Age of the affected animals: between 11 and 12 weeks.
- Percentage of dead pigs until the detection of the problem: 2 %.
- The affected animals had been vaccinated against *Mycoplasma hyopneumoniae* in the farrowing room (7 and 21 days) and had received their first vaccine against the Aujeszky's disease virus at 10 weeks of life.
- Zootechnical performance until the clinical outbreak: acceptable.

CLINICAL SIGNS OBSERVED

- The affected animals show pasty to watery diarrhoea of variable colour, with dark-yellowish faeces and reddish faeces due to the presence of fresh blood in the same batch of affected animals (Figs. 10, 11 and 12).
- The affected animals do not have a temperature but their general state progressively deteriorates.
- 18 % of the animals on the operation have similar signs.
- The mortality rate associated with this clinical problem is below 1 %.
- The clinical case has an average duration of 7 to 10 days in each sick animal. However,

the duration in the whole affected batch is longer than a month. This is due to the fact that new clinical cases appear progressively.

- At necropsy, a muco-haemorrhagic colitis and thickening of the mucosa at ileum near the ileocaecal junction are observed.

Differential diagnosis

The explanation of the procedures to reach a definitive diagnosis of each pathological process is out of the scope of this book. However, they will be discussed in depth in this case as it is essential to know the diagnostic process to understand how the antibiotic and the dosage regimen were chosen (Straw, 1999).

The diseases of the distal part of the small intestine and of the large intestine in pigs can be caused by several microorganisms. Next is a list of the aetiological agents that are most commonly involved as well as the name of the disease they cause:

1. Swine dysentery, whose aetiological agent is *Brachyspira hyodysenteriae* (BH).
2. Porcine intestinal spirochetosis (PIS), whose aetiological agent is *Brachyspira pilosicoli* (BP).
3. Porcine intestinal adenomatosis (PIA) or "proliferative ileitis", whose aetiological agent is *Lawsonia intracellularis* (LI).
4. Proliferative hemorrhagic enteropathy (PHE), whose aetiological agent is *Lawsonia intracellularis*. (LI).
5. Salmonellosis, whose aetiological agent is *Salmonella* spp (Spp).

Mixed infections are frequently found under field conditions. That is why it is essential to know the microorganism(s) involved in the clinical case. The use of pathological studies and laboratory techniques (PCR) that can detect the microorganism in faeces and/or the intestine are therefore recommended in order to reach an accurate diagnosis. It is very important to combine several techniques since pathogen excretion through faeces is mostly intermittent. Next is a summary of how the diagnosis was carried out.

STUDIES CARRIED OUT FOR THE DIAGNOSIS

Anatomopathological studies

- A complete necropsy of 3 pigs with typical clinical signs was performed. The pathological studies revealed the following:
  - In the ileum, caecum and colon of 3 animals:
    - Mild to moderate mononuclear colitis in the three animals.
    - Immunohistochemistry for the detection of LI. The result was positive in one of the three animals.
    - Warthin-Starry stain for the detection of spirochaetes (BH and BP). Two of the three animals gave a positive result.
  - Lung, lymph nodes, liver and kidney:
    - No apparent lesions.

In summary, inflammation can be observed in the colon of the affected animals and spirochaetes have been detected in the large intestine using a specific stain. Therefore, it seems reasonable to say that the clinical case is probably caused by *Brachyspira hyodysenteriae* and/or *Brachyspira pilosicoli* at the level of the large intestine. Moreover, *Lawsonia intracellularis* is responsible for the lesion observed in the distal part of the small intestine.

Molecular biology techniques of antigen detection (PCR)

- The following samples were taken and the following molecular biology techniques were applied:
  - Faeces of three necropsied animals (1 pool, P1).
  - Faeces of ten more animals that presented with the typical clinical picture (3 pools, P2, P3 and P4).
  - PCRs for the detection of BH, BP, Spp and LI (Table 5).

In summary, the presence of *Lawsonia intracellularis*, *Brachyspira hyodysenteriae* and *Brachyspira pilosicoli* in the faeces was confirmed by molecular biology techniques.

Interpretation of the pathological and antigen detection results

- The lesions at necropsy are compatible with swine dysentery and ileitis.
- The pathological studies point out that:
  - The lesions are compatible with swine dysentery as well as with porcine intestinal spirochaetosis.
  - There are lesions compatible with porcine intestinal adenomatosis in the ileum.
  - Spirochaetal bacteria are present.
- The molecular biology studies indicate:
  - presence of DNA from BH, BP and LI.
  - absence of DNA from Spp.

Therefore, the results indicate that the aetiological agents responsible for the clinical case are *Brachyspira hyodysenteriae* and *Lawsonia intracellularis*. However, the presence of *Brachyspira pilosicoli* has also been detected by molecular biology techniques. In this case, the animals may also be suffering from porcine intestinal spirochaetosis masked by the presence of swine dysentery.

In conclusion, the therapy will aim at controlling and/or eradicating *Brachyspira hyodysenteriae* and *Lawsonia intracellularis* on this farm. As previously discussed, an accurate diagnosis should be established before starting any treatment with antimicrobials. This statement can be extended to any therapy, but it is crucial in clinical cases such as the one we have just described, in which mixed infections are highly probable (Burch, 2005).

Brief description of swine dysentery

Swine dysentery (SD) is a severe muco-haemorrhagic colitis arising from the colonisation of the large intestine of pigs by *Brachyspira hyodysenteriae* (Hampson, 2006). These bacteria infect the large intestine and are excreted only through faeces. These anaerobic microorganisms inhabit the surface of the mucosa and, in addition, damage the cells of the mucosa. Furthermore, they can also penetrate the crypts of the large intestine (Fig. 13) and cause cellular necrosis and colitis. Susceptible animals can get infected by other animals (carrier mothers and gilts and affected animals) or the environment. The condition is seen mainly in grower or finisher pigs and less commonly in weaners. The disease is transmitted exclusively by faecal-oral route. The faeces are initially pasty and followed by abundant diarrhoea with very soft or liquid faeces containing mucus and undigested food. In some pigs, the faeces do not contain blood while in others, either from the beginning or after two or three days, the diarrhoea becomes bloody with a reddish to dark colour according to whether the animal is young or older. As the disease progresses, the faeces contain less blood, their colour can have a grey tone and they frequently carry plenty of tiny pieces of necrosed intestinal epithelium. Since the type, intensity and duration of the diarrhoea can greatly vary and the disease does not appear in all animals at the same time, it is possible at a given time to observe all the clinical forms of this enteric disease in the herd. This condition causes severe clinical problems and growth delays as well as an increase in the conversion index and in the production costs and in general, the reduction of the economic performance on the farm (Hampson, 2006).

A recent study concluded that SD is a major cause of diarrhoea in pigs of all ages raised on commercial farms in Spain (Carvajal, 2006). *Brachyspira hyodysenteriae* was identified in 32 % of the farms studied and in12 % of the faecal specimens collected from commercial pig farms with clinical signs of diarrhoea. Due to the lack of commercial vaccines, the control and treatment of SD involves the use of antimicrobials (Hampson, 2006). However, the control of SD has become complicated due to the emergence of strains with a reduced susceptibility to one or more of these antimicrobials, which has been recently reported in several countries (Molnar, 1996; Karlsson, 2001, 2003; Lobova, 2004; Rohde, 2004). As a result, careful use of the limited range of effective drugs currently available is now recommended (Karlsson, 2002), and the monitoring of resistance in clinical isolates of *Brachyspira hyodysenteriae* has become highly desirable (Karlsson, 2002; Rohde, 2004).

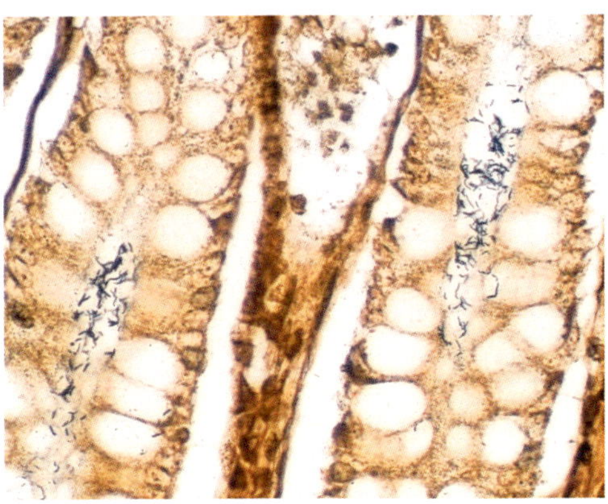

Figure 13

Brief description of ileitis (proliferative enteropathy)

Proliferative enteropathy (PE) is one of the most prevalent enteric bacterial diseases in grower and finisher pigs. *Lawsonia intracellularis* is an obligate intracellular bacterium that can only be cultivated and maintained in cell cultures (Nathues, 2009). This bacterium produces a common intestinal infection in pigs of economic significance in the pig industry worldwide (Jacobson, 2010). Pigs may under some circumstances become infected with LI with no reduction in the average daily gain (ADG) (Hybschmann, 2011). The clinical signs associated with the different intestinal pathogens are similar and microbiological investigations are necessary to confirm the specific microbiological cause in cases of diarrhoea. For LI, obtaining a correct microbiological diagnosis is complicated. Subclinical infection is common (McOrist, 2005) and LI can be demonstrated by PCR in animals vaccinated with an avirulent live vaccine. Later on, pigs can potentially shed detectable numbers of LI in faeces for 8 to 12 weeks (Smith, 1997). Demonstration of LI in the faeces is therefore not necessarily associated with a clinical problem such as uneven growth in a group of pigs. The bacterial load in faeces could not be assessed using routine diagnostic tests in the past as the bacterium could only be cultivated and maintained in cell cultures. Development of quantitative PCR (qPCR) tests for the quantification of LI in faeces (Nathues, 2009; Richter, 2010; Stahl, 2011) has now made it possible to determine the number of bacteria in faeces on a routine basis. This may be useful for confirmation of LI as the microbiological cause of porcine diarrhoea. It has recently been demonstrated that the average *Lawsonia intracellularis* excretion was significantly higher in pigs with gross lesions of proliferative enteropathy (average excretion: 5.92 log10 bacteria/g faeces) than in pigs without gross lesions of proliferative enteropathy (average excretion: < 3.3 log10 bacteria/g faeces) (Petersen, 2012). Increasing numbers of LI log10 bacteria/g faeces were significantly associated with a decreasing average daily gain (Petersen, 2012). The treatment of a PE outbreak on a pig farm often involves antimicrobial therapy.

Initial treatment

Symptomatic

The animals ate feed in pellets with a standard formula for their age. After confirming the diagnosis of swine dysentery as part of the aetiology of this clinical case, the animals were given feed in meal form and rice was included in the feed (10 % of the total amount of raw materials). Obviously, the composition of the new formula also covered the animals' nutritional needs.

Aetiologic

Administration of an antibiotic following the manufacturer's specifications. The parenteral and oral routes can be used in the most and least affected animals respectively. This point will be discussed in depth further on.

CRITICAL REVIEW OF THE TREATMENTS

Therapeutic approach

Symptomatic

The influence of diet on the clinical presentation of digestive diseases in general and swine dysentery in particular has been greatly discussed. As previously explained, the feed administered to the animals after the diagnosis of the disease was in meal form and rice was included in its composition (10 % of the total amount of the feed raw materials). This nutritional strategy can be used in pig production for the "treatment" of this disease (Fraile, personal communication) and it is supported by scientific studies (Pluske, 1996). That is to say, when planning the treatment of digestive diseases, it is not only necessary to design therapeutic programmes with antimicrobials, but it is also worth working together with the nutritionist to achieve a more efficient resolution of the clinical and performance problem.

Aetiologic

When deciding on an antimicrobial treatment for this disease, it is essential to identify the objective we aim to achieve: avoiding the appearance of the disease or treating a clinical outbreak that has already taken place. In any case, antibiotic treatments will have to be administered to a very large number of animals. Therefore, the most frequent route of administration will be the oral route (mainly through feed). That is why we should focus on the oral route of administration in the optimisation of the dosage regimen, although we will also discuss the use of the intramuscular route for those animals at a more advanced clinical stage. In addition, the intramuscular route will also be taken into account since it could also be used as a tool in the treatment of this disease and even in eradication programmes (Szancer, 2005).

CRITICAL REVIEW OF THE ADMINISTRATION OF ANTIBIOTICS IN THE TREATMENT

Need to use antibiotics

There is a generalised consensus in the literature on the need to use antibiotics when designing a therapy in clinical cases of swine dysentery and ileitis (Prescott, 2000). Fortunately, there are antibiotics available that have shown to be effective for the treatment of these diseases. Indeed, it is possible to use antibiotics that belong to the class of lincosamides (lincomycin), macrolides (tylvalosin and tylosin) and pleuromutilins (tiamulin and valnemulin).

The possible use of spectinomycin in the treatment of ileitis will be reviewed in combination with the administration of lincomycin.

Therapeutic approach

In the case of swine dysentery and ileitis, the therapeutic approach is the following:

- The infection is mainly located in the large intestine (dysentery) and the distal part of the small intestine (ileitis).
- The dosage regimen should be chosen according to the therapeutic objective that has been set. This objective can either be preventing the appearance of the disease (prevention) or treating the infection once the animals already present with the clinical picture.
- The chosen dosage regimen must reach a sufficient concentration at the site of action (in this case, the large intestine for dysentery and the distal part of the small intestine for ileitis) so it can inhibit bacterial growth and be maintained for a sufficient period of time.
- The concentration that must be attained will depend on the clinical evolution of the animals. It is very different if the disease is recent or if it has been established for a long time.
- The infection is chronic. Therefore, the treatments must be of long duration.

PHARMACODYNAMIC PROPERTIES

An antibiotic should be chosen taking into account the following considerations. In this case, the first point to be analysed is that the antimicrobial should be active against BH and LI. As explained in the first chapter, antimicrobial susceptibility against BH is usually measured with the MIC value. The MIC values (following standardised methods for their determination) of a list of antimicrobials that may be used in a BH outbreak are shown in Table 6 and Figure 14.

Finally, antimicrobial susceptibility against LI is also measured with the MIC value. LI is an intracellular microorganism and determination of the MIC values for this pathogen has peculiarities that must be briefly discussed. Although methodologies for determining antimicrobial sensitivity of intracellular organisms have been developed, the methods and interpretation of their results have not been standardised or uniformly accepted. Thus, the extracellular and intracellular MIC values for LI are usually determined by trying to mimic LI infections in which the bacteria are exposed to antimicrobials before and after invasion of the intestinal cells. The extracellular and intracellular MICs of various antimicrobials against a number of isolates of LI has been described in the literature (McOrist, 1995) and these values were determined when the inhibition by the antimicrobials was greater than 99 %. The extracellular MIC value was determined by adding antimicrobials to a medium with LI, which was used to infect a cell culture. After 24 hours, the culture medium was replaced with a fresh medium without antimicrobials. However, the intracellular MIC was determined in a rat intestinal epithelial cell culture infected with LI, and the total duration of the antibiotic treatment at several concentrations was 72 hours. The medium was then replaced until day seven with non-medicated medium. In both cases (extracellular and intracellular MIC values), the cell cultures were examined to count the number of bacteria inside the cells. A heavily infected cell (HIC) was defined as a cell containing more than 30 LI. The results were expressed as the percentage of HICs in treated cultures divided by the mean HICs in untreated cultures to give a percentage of inhibition due to the antibiotic.

The MIC values of a list of antimicrobials that may be used in an LI outbreak can be found

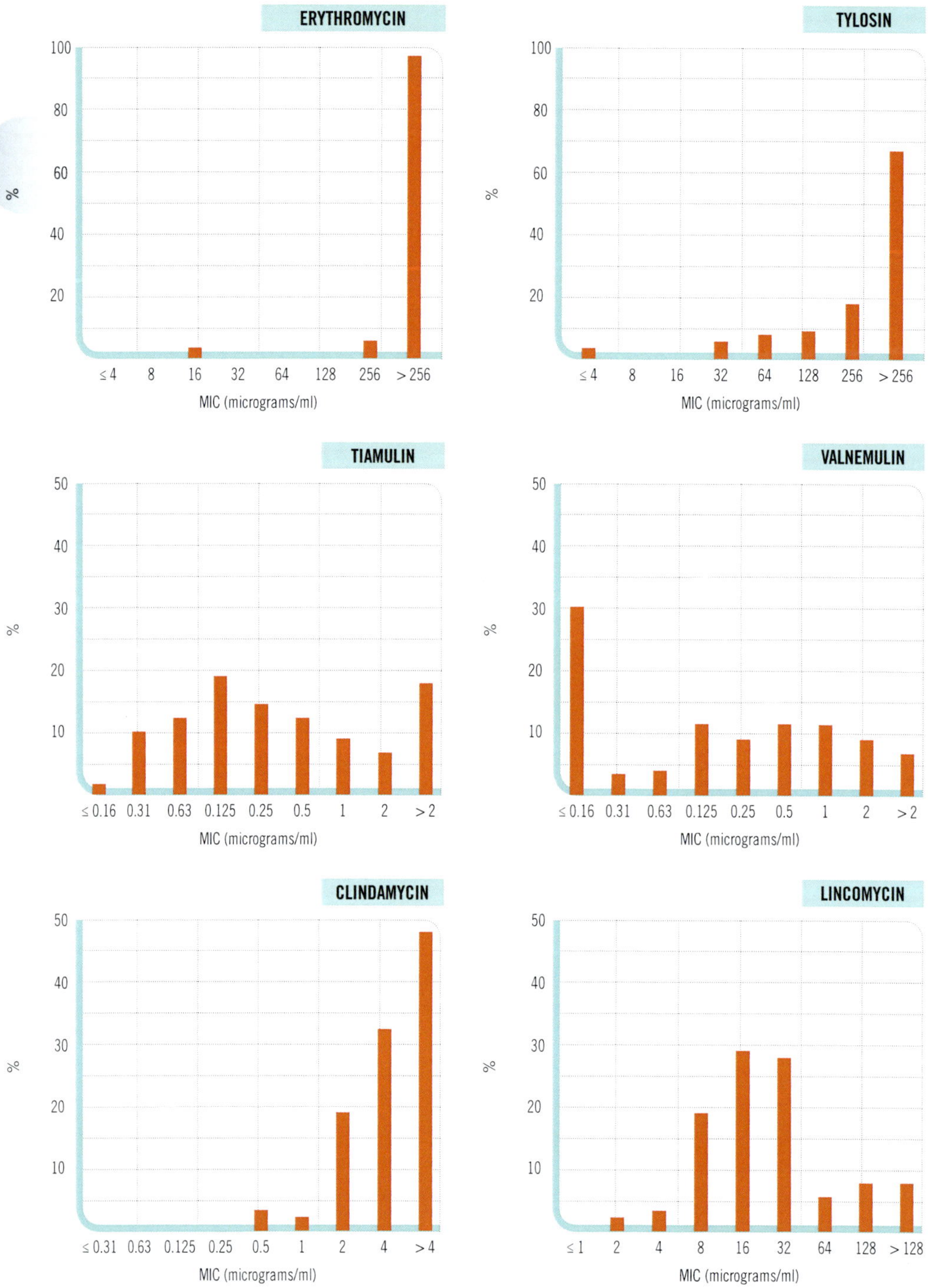

Figure 14. MIC values of six antimicrobial agents for 108 Spanish field isolates of *B. hyodysenteriae* recovered between 2000 and 2007.

in Table 7. It should be highlighted that the number of isolates available to carry out these determinations was low due to the difficulty to isolate these bacteria.

PHARMACOKINETIC PROPERTIES

The second element that needs to be known is the concentration of the antimicrobial that will be reached at the site of action. In this case, the site of action is the intestine and more precisely the contents of the colon for BH and the contents of the ileum and its mucosa for LI. Tables 8 and 9 show the penetration of the antimicrobials that may be used to treat a BH and LI outbreak at this site depending on their inclusion rate in the feed.

Pleuromutilins, valnemulin and tiamulin appear to achieve relatively low concentrations in the ileum in comparison with lincomycin and tylosin. Acetylisovaleryltylosin achieves a concentration that is in-between those of pleuromutilins and lincosamides.

PECULIARITIES OF THE TREATMENT OF DIGESTIVE DISEASES

Studies on antimicrobial use in digestive diseases are aimed at defining the most appropriate dosage regimen either for the prevention or for treatment of these clinical entities. Preventive treatments can be defined as those that are applied to prevent the clinical appearance of the disease and curative treatments as those that are applied after the clinical signs have appeared.

It is easy to see in the summary of product characteristics that the doses used in preventive programmes are much lower than those used in therapeutic programmes (preventive/treatment ratio of 1:2-3). One of the reasons that can explain these different dosages lies in the fact that in healthy animals, the drug directly penetrates the crypts to exert its effect, while in sick animals the drug must penetrate the crypts and pass through several layers of mucus and exudate, fibrin and cellular debris. Another reason that can explain this difference is that animals suffering from digestive diseases have a lower feed intake and the concentration of the drug in feed must therefore be increased to compensate for this factor. It should be pointed out that the microorganism can be eradicated (bacteriological cure) with the preventive programme. Indeed, a dose-response effect for prevention and treatment can be observed (Figs. 15 and 16). In both cases, elimination of the bacteria can be achieved. Therefore, it is not possible to argue that lower doses in the case of preventive programmes could increase the appearance of resistances. This point is very relevant because, for other diseases, the doses used for preventive purposes should be the same as those used for treatment (e.g. tulathromycin in the porcine respiratory disease complex).

These data highlight the fact that the objective of the therapy must be known (prevention vs. treatment) before starting the treatment, and that using lower doses without taking into account the goal previously mentioned is not justifiable. Unfortunately, in clinical practice lower doses than those recommended by laboratories are sometimes used for economic reasons only. Yet it is easy to understand that if the doses recommended for preventive programmes are used for the treatment of clinical cases that are "not very severe" (but in which the disease is already established), it is very likely that the treatment will not be effective and, in addition, the probability of the appearance of bacterial resistances is increased.

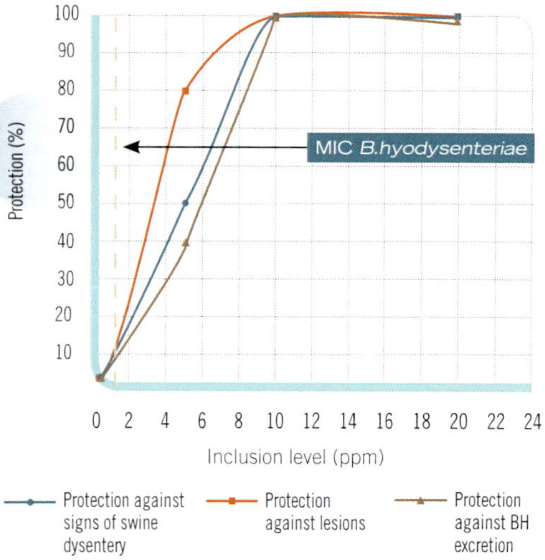

Figure 15. Protection against signs of swine dysentery, lesions due to BH infection and excretion of BH depending on the antibiotic concentration used in the feed to prevent the appearance of the disease.

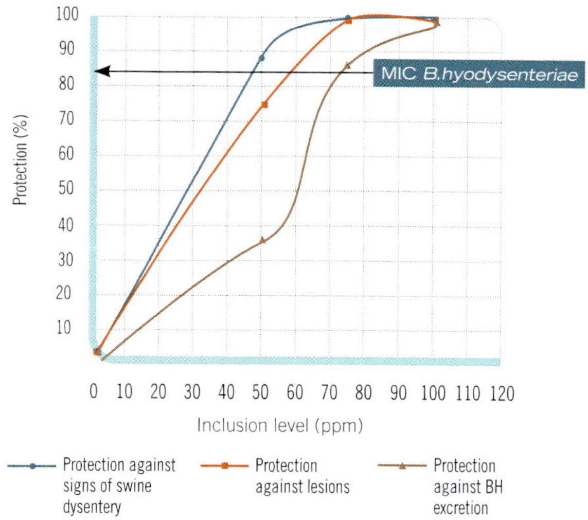

Figure 16. Protection against swine dysentery symptoms, lesions due to BH infection and excretion of BH depending on the antibiotic concentration used in the feed for affected animals (treatment).

INTEGRATION OF PK AND PD INFORMATION

Much of the work in humans and animals to integrate pharmacokinetic and pharmacodynamic information has focused on concentration-dependent, bactericidal and injectable antimicrobials such as fluoroquinolones to treat respiratory diseases. However, very little PK/PD modelling work has been reported for primarily bacteriostatic antimicrobials administered orally, mainly in feed, to treat major gut infections in pigs such as ileitis (porcine intestinal adenomatosis) and swine dysentery. Even less information is available when these antibiotics are administered by parenteral route. The information about PK and PD integration will be explained next depending on the route of administration:

Oral administration

The PK/PD parameters of the antimicrobials that may be used should be calculated for each clinical case in order to predict clinical efficacy in a case by case situation. As an example, the PK/PD parameters of a time-dependent antibiotic (lincomycin) in the case of swine dysentery and ileitis when this antibiotic is administered by oral route are given next.

LINCOMYCIN AND SWINE DYSENTERY

In prevention studies, the antibiotic is administered before, during, or soon after the infection, before clinical signs have appeared and some colonisation may have occurred, whereas treatment is administered when there are clinical signs or shedding of the organism is occurring, usually 7-21 days after infection. With treatment trials, there is usually a treatment period of 7-21 days, followed by an observation period of 2-3 weeks, to determine whether the disease has been eliminated and the organism completely destroyed or whether recrudescence occurs. This is usually confirmed by necrospy and culture of the colon. In prevention studies, there are sometimes no follow-up observation periods and necrospy may be performed at the end of the trial. This may mean that the organism is not completely eliminated, but inhibited to such an extent that it does not cause any visible gross lesions, and may be present below the limit for detection or recovery by culture.

From the studies available in the literature (Duhamel, 1997), it can be concluded that the colonic concentrations (CC) of lincomycin should be closer to the MIC (CC/MIC ratio around 1) in order to be effective either for preventive or treatment purposes. In other words, lincomycin behaves as a time-dependent antibiotic when it is chosen to treat BH infections. Moreover, in some cases, this ratio is lower than the MIC value (0.51) and the treatment is still effective. For this reason, other factors may play a role that justifies the efficacy observed under field conditions when lincomycin is the chosen antibiotic. It has been hypothesised that lincomycin may have an effect on other bacteria present in the colon. Indeed, it has recently been reported that antibiotic treatments in pigs significantly modify the microbioma of this part of the intestine (Looft, 2012). This modification may have a significant effect on the final outcome of the treatment but this hypothesis should be verified experimentally.

The PK/PD parameter linked with clinical efficacy for lincomycin is in absolute contrast with that described for pleuromutilins (tiamulin and valnemulin). In the case of pleuromutilins (tiamulin and valnemulin), colonic concentration/MBC ratios of at least 18 and 180 must be achieved to cause complete growth inhibition of BH in a prevention study and to eliminate the infection, respectively (Burch, 2005). However, the PK/PD parameter linked with clinical efficacy for lincomycin is T > MIC.

LINCOMYCIN USED FOR ILEITIS PREVENTION OR TREATMENT

In a study conducted by Winkelman (1999), an infectious challenge model was used to study the possible use of lincomycin in the prevention of porcine ileitis. Pigs were medicated for 4 days prior to infection and for a further 31 days with lincomycin at 0 (control group), 44 and 110 ppm and tylosin at 110 ppm as another control treatment. The trial was ended and the pigs necropsied on day 35. The results obtained can be observed in Table 10.

The mortality rate was very high in the untreated control group, which demonstrates the severity of the challenge. The lesion was also long in the controls groups, but it was significantly reduced by lincomycin at 44 and 110 ppm, although, surprisingly, little difference was observed between the two doses. These results were confirmed by merging data from a previous study following the same experimental design (Winkelman et al., 1998; Winkelman, 1999). The global results are summarised in Table 11.

This can be considered a relatively aggressive model, as the mortality was 52 % in the untreated controls, whereas in field infections it is considerably lower. It can be considered as a severe challenge infection model and the results obtained are probably those of a worst-case scenario.

The gut pharmacokinetics of lincomycin can be correlated with its inhibitory effect on *Lawsonia intracellularis* in vitro and linked with data from clinical trials. A clear dose-response effect can be observed between the ileal concentrations for 110, 44 and 22 ppm in feed and the intracellular (IC) and extracellular (EC) inhibition curves for lincomycin (Fig. 17). In conclusion, a PK/PD model can be established in the treatment of LI infections. The IC/EC inhibitory concentration may be considered too restrictive at 99 % inhibition, as a good clinical effect may be achieved at lower levels of, for example, 90 %. Thus, in Figure 17, it can be observed that a percentage of inhibition of 90 and 99 % is achieved with an ileal lincomycin concentration of 12 and 32 µg/ml, respectively. Linking it with the dose administered in feed, both 44 and 110 ppm would be expected to exert a marked inhibitory effect (greater than 90 % inhibition) against LI contained intracellularly. However, 22 ppm would not be so effective for treatment but could exert a good preventative effect on extracellular organisms (Burch, 2003).

The effect of different doses of lincomycin on performance (ADG and FCE) and disease (mortality and lesion length) can also be analysed in order to try to correlate them with the intracellular and extracellular inhibition effects of the different lincomycin concentrations determined in vitro. Figure 18 shows that, in terms of disease prevention, the mortality and inhibition figures were the most similar. Both curves seemed to plateau at 44 ppm and there were minor movements up and down at 110 ppm. Curiously, lincomycin at 22 ppm was able to obtain a marked reduction in mortality but without reaching the same results as those observed for higher doses. Finally, performance characteristics (ADG and FCE) improved significantly at 22 ppm and reached a plateau at 44 ppm. One major issue with any antibiotic treatment is the appearance of bacterial resistance. It has been described that a risk factor for its development is the use of low doses of antibiotics. In this sense, (McOrist, personal communication) the generation of antimicrobial resistance for this bacteria is highly unlikely since the generation of resistant bacteria is an energy dependent processes and these mechanisms are not available in this type of special intracellular bacteria.

Lincomycin showed a lower efficacy in early treatment probably due to the internalisation of the organism into the cell, which takes about three hours (Gebhart, 2004). However, spectinomycin showed a marked improvement in early treatment, presumably because it has a higher bactericidal activity against the unprotected organism and poor cell penetration. In general terms, spectinomycin mainly acts on extracellular LI whereas lincomycin mainly acts on LI in the cell. For this reason, lincomycin is usually combined with spectinomycin to treat

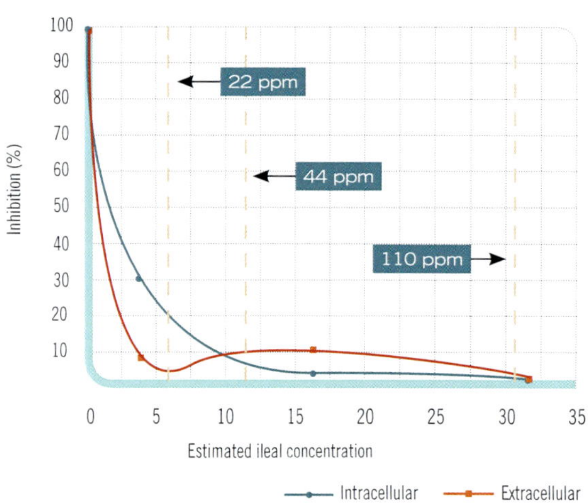

Figure 17. Intracellular and extracellular inhibition curves for lincomycin against *L. intracellularis* plus estimated ileal concentrations for 110, 44 and 22 ppm in feed.

ileitis due to the clear synergic effect of this combination in the treatment of an LI infection.

Table 12 shows the probability of clinical success for the antimicrobials that may used for the treatment of BH and LI infections, calculated taking into account the pharmacokinetic and pharmacodynamic data provided by the pharmaceutical companies or available in the public domain.

The information provided in Table 12 is for guidance only, since each strain has its own MIC value for each antimicrobial. The PK/PD parameters of the antimicrobials that may be used should therefore be calculated for each clinical case and the result should be taken into account to optimise the therapy and choose the best antimicrobial option (see Fig. 14 in chapter 2). In addition, in order to choose an appropriate antimicrobial agent, swine practitioners should know the efficacy of the molecule (previously analysed), the current regulations on the use of antimicrobials in their country and the history of the herd.

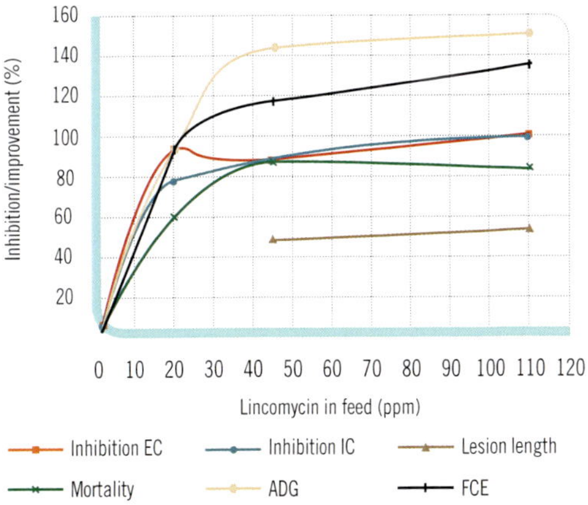

Figure 18. Predictive inhibition and actual effect of lincomycin included in the feed at 22, 44 and 110 ppm.

Parenteral route

In this clinical case, it was also necessary to administer antibiotics by intramuscular route to the animals with very severe clinical symptoms for a period of time. In this specific case, the administration of antibiotics by intramuscular route is indicated in the treatment of swine dysentery since these animals have a very low feed intake and the administration of antibiotics mixed with feed does not seem to be the best route of administration. However, the intramuscular administration of drugs in pigs implies extra work and reduces animal welfare. As previously discussed, this infection is chronic and requires the administration of antibiotics for long periods of time. If we take this information into consideration, it is easy to understand that the intramuscular administration of antibiotics for 3 days may control the clinical signs but will probably not eradicate the microorganism from the affected animals. That is why a common approach is to combine parenteral therapy (in the most affected animals) with oral therapy for the least affected animals and those that have started to improve clinically with parenteral therapy.

The administration of a drug by parenteral route in the treatment of a gastrointestinal disease always raises the issue of whether the drug will reach the site of action (digestive tract) in the sufficient amount to exert its effect. Unfortunately, there is little information about the penetration of antibiotics in the digestive tract after parenteral administration and there are also no PK/PD studies available for these drugs when they are administered by intramuscular route in the treatment of swine dysentery and ileitis. Although there are no PK/PD studies available, the efficacy of the treatment is supported by the clinical trials pharmaceutical laboratories carried out when they applied for the authorisation of new antibiotics by intramuscular route for this indication.

Final observations on the treatment of digestive diseases

All the people involved in swine production know that, on quite a few occasions, the treatment of digestive diseases is frustrating because the objectives are not reached. It would be necessary to answer the following questions before considering making any changes in the therapeutic programme that was initially designed:

1. Has the diagnosis been carried out correctly? We have already seen that on many occasions, there are cases of mixed infections that make the design of a therapeutic programme more difficult.
2. Does the feed given to the animals contain the required amount of antibiotic? This is a critical point and a frequent cause of failures in the treatment.
3. Are the animals eating the theoretical amount of feed? This is a critical point since doses are based on theoretical intakes, which are hardly verified under field conditions.
4. Has the MIC value been determined for the microorganism or has it been assumed that it does not differ significantly from the value normally reported in the population?

Table 1. MIC of antimicrobials for the treatment of *Escherichia coli* infections (Burch, 2007).

Antimicrobial	MIC range (μg/ml)	MIC_{90} (μg/ml)	Epidemiological cut-off (μg/ml)	Clinical cut-off (μg/ml)
Danofloxacin	0.03-1	0.125	-	-
Enrofloxacin	0.03-1	0.25	0.06	2
Ampicillin	1-64	64	8	16
Amoxicillin + clavulanic acid	2-64	8	16	16
Sulfamethoxazole + Trimethoprim	0.5-8	8	1	4
Sulfadiazine + Trimethoprim	0.31- > 40	1.25*	-	-
Neomycin	2-64	64	4	8
Spectinomycin	8-256	256	32	64
Colistin sulphate	2-4	2	4	8

* MIC_{50}

Table 2. Penetration of antimicrobials in the intestinal content after parenteral administration.

Antimicrobial group	Example	Penetration at the site of action	Reference
Fluoroquinolones	Marbofloxacin Danofloxacin	++/+++	Baggot et al., 2000
β-lactam antibiotics	Amoxicillin	+	
Cephalosporins	Ceftiofur	+	
Sulphonamides	Sulfadimethoxine	+	

-, no, + low, ++ intermediate and +++ high penetration.

Table 3. PK/PD parameters calculated for danofloxacin in the treatment of EC infections in different parts of the intestine.

Parameter	Intestinal content (ic)	Mucosa of the small intestine (m)
AUCic/MIC	432	-
AUCm/MIC	-	581
Cmax/MIC	15.28	38.96

Table 4. Probability of clinical success for antimicrobials in the treatment of EC infections.

Antimicrobial group	Example	PK/PD parameter and threshold value	Probability of success
Fluoroquinolones	Marbofloxacin Danofloxacin	Cmax/MIC > 10 and AUC/MIC > 100	+++
Cephalosporins	Ceftiofur	T > MIC	+/++
Sulphonamides	Sulfadiazine	T > MIC	-/+
Sulphonamides + Diaminopyrimidines	Sulfadiazine + Trimethoprim	T > MIC	+/++
Aminoglycosides	Neomycin	Cmax/MIC > 10	+++
Amynocyclitols	Spectinomycin	T > MIC	+/++
Polymyxins	Colistin sulphate	Cmax/MIC and AUC/MIC	+++

Probability of success: - failure, + low, ++ intermediate and +++ high.

Table 5. PCR results of different pools coming from 13 animals showing similar signs in a clinical case (see text for abbreviations).

Pools of faeces	LI	BH	BP	Spp
P1	-	+	-	-
P2	+	-	-	-
P3	+	+	-	-
P4	+	+	+	-

Table 6. MIC of antimicrobials for the treatment of a BH infection.

	Hidalgo et al., 2011 (Spain)		Pringle et al., 2012 (Sweden)	
Antimicrobial	**MIC range (µg/ml)**	**MIC_{90} (µg/ml)**	**MIC range (µg/ml)**	**MIC_{90} (µg/ml)**
Lincomycin	1- > 64	> 64	0.5- > 64	32
Tiamulin	0.063- > 8	8	0.016-1	0.25
Valnemulin	0.031- > 4	4	0.031-0.5	0.063
Tylosin	16- > 128	> 128	2- > 128	> 128
Tylvalosin	0.5- > 32	16	0.25- > 32	16

Table 7. MIC of antimicrobials for the treatment of a LI infection.

	Burch, 2005 (2 or 3 isolates)		Wattanaphansak et al., 2009 (10 isolates from USA and Denmark)	
Antimicrobial	**Intracellular MIC range (µg/ml)**	**Extracellular MIC_{90} (µg/ml)**	**Intracellular MIC range (µg/ml)**	**Extracellular MIC_{90} (µg/ml)**
Lincomycin	32	32	8- > 128	32- > 128
Tiamulin	4	4	0.125-0.5	1-32
Valnemulin	< 2	-	0.125	0.125-4
Tylosin	64	64	0.5-8	1- > 128
Spectinomycin*	32	32	ND	ND

ND not determined.

*One strain.

Table 8. Concentration in colonic contents (µg/g) of various antibiotics at different feed levels (ppm).

Antibiotic / Concentration	**Levels in feed (ppm) / Concentrations in colon (µg/g)**		
Valnemulin	200	75	25
Concentration	**5.2**	**1.68**	**0.56-0.65 (0.61) E**
Tiamulin	220	110	44
Concentration	**8.05**	**2.84**	**1.12-1.61 (1.37) E**
Lincomycin	220	110	44
Concentration	**101**	**34.5**	**13.8-20.2 (17.0) E**
Tylosin	200	100	40
Concentration	**100 E**	**50 E**	**20 E**
Acetylisovaleryltylosin	200	100	50
Concentration	**> 10-35 (22.5) E**	**> 5-17.5 (11.3) E**	**> 2.5-8.8 (5.5) E**

E: estimate; proportionately related to reported values.

Table 9. Concentration in ileal contents of various antibiotics at different feed levels.

Antibiotic / Concentration	**Levels in feed (ppm) / Concentrations in ileum (µg/g)**		
Valnemulin	200	75	25
Concentration	**1.51**	**0.49**	**0.17-0.19 (0.18) E**
Tiamulin	220	110	44
Concentration	**2.33**	**0.82**	**0.32-.047 (0.40) E**
Lincomycin	220	110	44
Concentration	**29.29**	**10.01**	**4.0-5.86 (4.93) E**
Tylosin	200	100	40
Concentration	**29 E**	**14.5 E**	**5.8 E**
Acetylisovaleryltylosin	200	100	50
Concentration	**> 2.9-10.15 (6.53) E**	**> 1.45-5.08 (3.28) E**	**> 0.73-2.55 (1.60) E**

E: estimate; proportionately related to reported values.

Table 10. Efficacy of lincomycin and tylosin for the prevention of ileitis.

Treatment group (ppm)	**Mortality (%)**	**Intestinal lesion length (cm)**
Lincomycin 0	52	160 (-)
Lincomycin 44	4	84 (-48 %)*
Lincomycin 110	12	79 (-51 %)*
Tylosin 110	16	109 (-32 %)

*p = < 0.05

Table 11. Results for lincomycin in feed in a prevention study.

Treatment (ppm)	ADG (g)	FCE	Lesion length (cm)	Mortality (%)
Untreated infected control	95	0.18	160	52
Lincomycin 22	182	0.35	NR	20
Lincomycin 44	232	0.39	84	4
Lincomycin 110	241	0.42	79	8
Tylosin 110	168	0.32	109	16

Table 12. Probability of clinical success for antimicrobials in the treatment of BH and LI infections.

Antimicrobial	PK/PD parameter	Probability of success for BH treatment	Probability of success for LI treatment
Lincomycin	T > MIC	++/+++	+++
Tiamulin	CC/MIC and AUC/MIC	++/+++	++/+++
Valnemulin	CC/MIC and AUC/MIC	+++	+++
Tylosin	T > MIC	-	+++
Spectinomycin	T > MIC	-	+++*

Probability of success: - failure, + low, ++ intermediate and +++ high.

*Always combined with lincomycin for this purpose.

CC: colonic concentrations.

4 Treatment of meningitis and skin infections

Treatment of meningitis and skin infections

4

General concepts

As opposed to other chapters, the general physiopathological characteristics of meningitis and skin infections will not be reviewed here as they will be seen in the clinical cases studied.

Penetration of the antibiotic at the site of action

PENETRATION IN THE CENTRAL NERVOUS SYSTEM

As we have seen in the introductory chapter, pharmacokinetics enables us to predict the blood or plasma concentration of a drug after its administration, but it does not allow us to know the concentrations in the other tissues of the organism at the same kinetic times, unless tissue samples are also taken. As explained in previous chapters, it is important to know the tissue concentration because it is the concentration of antibiotic that is present in the target organ(s).

When establishing the treatment of an infection in the CNS, it is essential to know the drug concentration in this organ. The central nervous system is a very complex "organ". The diagram next (Fig. 1) represents the different "compartments" that exist from a pharmacological point of view. There are two "barriers" between the blood and the central nervous system. The first is the blood-brain barrier (BBB), which is formed by endothelial cells that are "tightly" joined and the second is a barrier that regulates the passage of the cerebrospinal fluid (blood-cerebrospinal fluid-barrier, B-CSF-B) which is

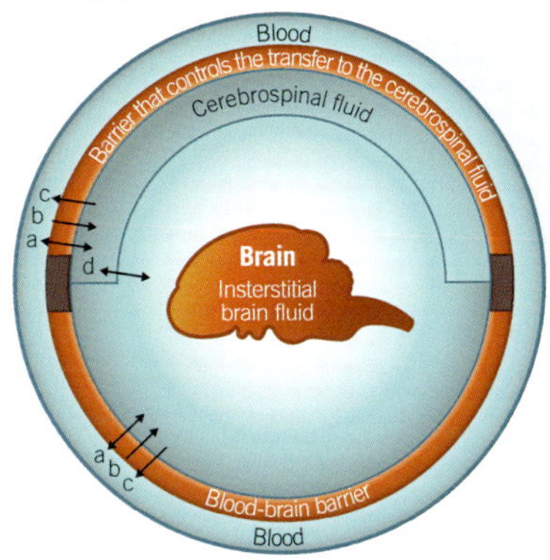

Figure 1. Representation of the different compartments available in the central nervous system from a pharmacological point of view.

formed by epithelial cells of the choroid plexus (De Lange, 2002; De Boer, 2003). These barriers delimit three compartments from a pharmacological point of view in the CNS: blood, cerebrospinal fluid and interstitial fluid (ISF). Figure 1 also represents the transport processes that exist in these barriers (De Lange, 2005):

a. Passive diffusion through a transcellular or paracellular route (represented as "a" in the figure).
b. Facilitated or active transport into the CNS mediated by receptors (represented as "b" in the figure).
c. Active transport out of the CNS (represented as "c" in the figure).
d. Passive diffusion between the brain interstitial fluid and the cerebrospinal fluid. In this case there are no cellular barriers with tight junctions (represented as "d" in the figure).

With the exception of the diseases that primarily affect the brain surface such as meningitis, it is more relevant to know the drug concentration in the brain tissue than in the cerebrospinal fluid (Partridge, 1988). However, it is much more usual to find information about the concentration in the latter because samples can easily be obtained from this compartment. It is usually only possible to find information such as that shown in Figure 2 for ceftriaxone (cephalosporin for humans).

It would be ideal to be able to distinguish between the drug concentration in the cerebral interstitial fluid and inside the cells (intracellular) as well as the concentration related to the cellular membranes in the brain tissue. This information is very difficult to obtain because of the methodological difficulties it entails. However, from a purely practical point of view, in veterinary medicine, the cases of meningoencephalitis that need to be treated with antimicrobials are of bacterial origin; therefore, the optimisation of their treatment does not require such deep knowledge of the concentrations in the different compartments (Van Bree, 1988).

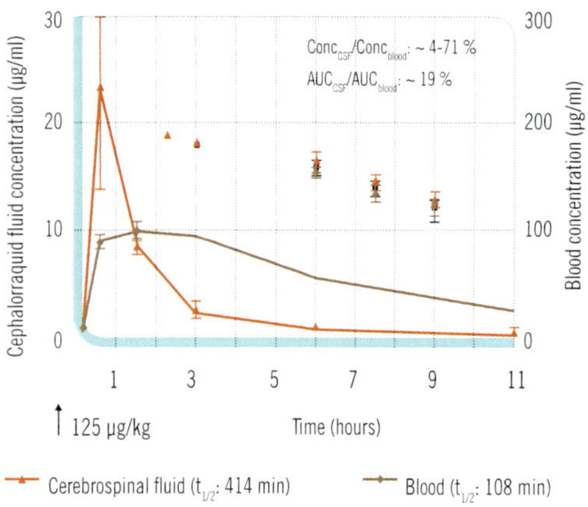

Figure 2. Ceftioxone concentration in blood and cerebrospinal fluid during therapy for pneumococcal meningitis in humans.

Conc$_{CSF}$/Conc$_{blood}$: ratio cerebrospinal fluid concentration/blood concentration.

AUC$_{CSF}$/AUC$_{blood}$: ratio AUC in cerebrospinal fluid and in blood.

Infections of the central nervous system are special when compared with infections in peripheral areas. For bacteria to invade the CNS, the blood-brain barrier must be damaged (Fig. 1). A deficiency in immunoglobulins, complement and leukocytes in the cerebrospinal fluid allows rapid bacterial growth. The defence mechanisms at the level of the CNS are limited. Therefore, in principle, only the antibiotics that reach bactericidal concentrations in the cerebrospinal fluid should be used in the treatment of meningitis (Dowling, 1999).

In principle, due to the existence of the blood-brain barrier, in order for antito reach therapeutic concentrations of antimicrobials in the CNS, these must be liposoluble, with low molecular weight, a low degree of binding to plasma proteins and they must be weak bases so they can concentrate due to the "ion-trapping" phenomenon at the level of the CNS (Oldendorf, 1974; Suzuki, 1997) (Fig. 3). However, when the blood-brain barrier is inflamed, its permeability is increased (Figs. 4a and 4b). This phenomenon explains why penicillins and cephalosporins (weak organic acids) accumulate in the CNS in case of inflammation (Bodor, 1982). The choice of antibiotics in the treatment of infections of the CNS must be based on the penetration of the antibiotic in this organ and on a presumptive diagnosis of the bacterium that must be treated (at least whether it is gram-positive or negative). Different types of antibiotics are classified according to their capacity to penetrate in the CNS in Table 1. However, this information is for guidance only since the real penetration of the drug in the CNS is substantially modified as a consequence of the inflammation of this organ and many of the basic studies are carried out only on healthy animals.

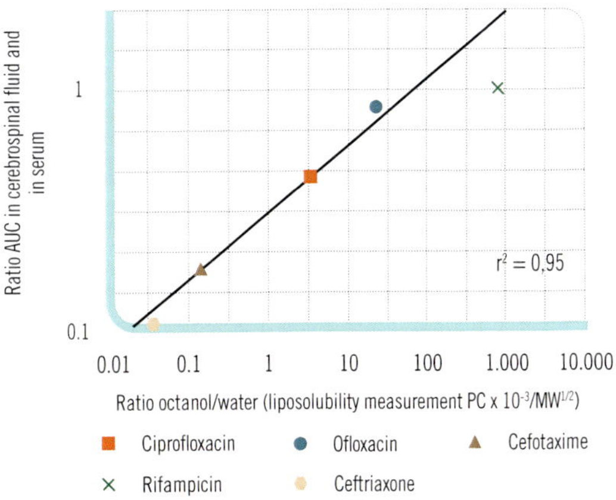

Figure 3. Penetration of antibiotics in the cerebrospinal fluid depending on their liposolubility (a higher liposolubility means a higher penetration). Nau, R. et al., J. Neurol. Sci., 1994.

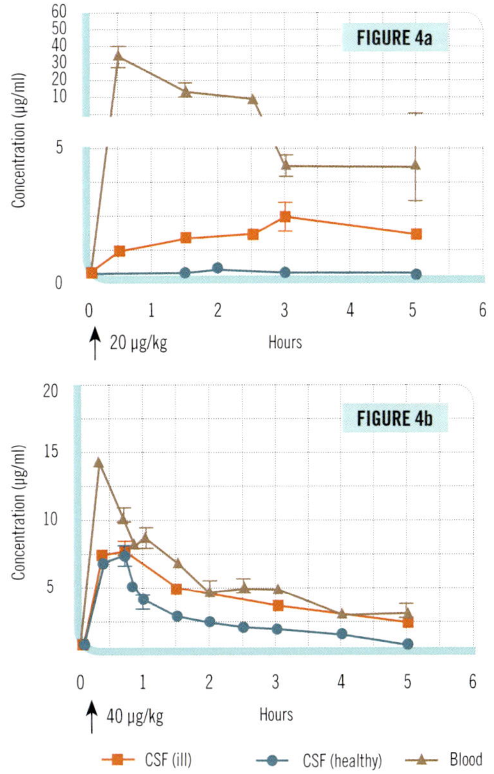

Figures 4a and 4b. Vancomycin (4a) and moxifloxacin (4b) concentrations in blood and cerebrospinal fluid in patients affected by meningitis and healthy patients.

CSF (ill) µg/ml: concentration in cerebrospinal fluid in patients affected by meningitis.
CSF (healthy) µg/ml: concentration in cerebrospinal fluid in healthy patients.

PENETRATION OF THE ANTIBIOTIC IN THE SKIN

The skin represents the anatomical limit and the limit of communication between the animal and its environment. It is a very heterogeneous organ that includes a variety of cellular and tissue components: the epidermis, a system of appendices, the dermis, the erector muscles of hair and a fat layer (subcutaneous fat). Describing all the diseases that can affect the skin as well as their treatment is beyond the aims of this book. In fact, it will be only described diseases in which bacterial microorganisms are involved in its pathogenesis and antimicrobials are therefore a key element in its therapy.

As we have seen in the introductory chapter, pharmacokinetics enables us to predict the blood or plasma concentration of a drug after its administration, but it does not allow us to know the concentrations in the other tissues of the organism at the same kinetic times, unless tissue samples are also taken. In cases of skin infections, we face the same problem. The fact that the antibiotic concentration in the different parts of the skin is not usually measured is another disadvantage. As we have previously explained, skin is a complex tissue and it would be interesting to know the penetration of the drug in the different segments.

There are no specific studies about the penetration of β-lactam antibiotics in the skin of species of veterinary interest. However, there is information available about the penetration of these antibiotics in skin abscesses in an experimental mouse model. As can be seen in Figure 5, imipenem (which also belongs to the β-lactam family of antibiotics) reaches a higher concentration in abscesses than in plasma throughout the whole treatment. In addition, the penetration of other β-lactam drugs in "subcutaneous tissue cages" is sufficient to control the infection by *Streptococcus zooepidermicus* in ponies (Ensink, 1996) and to prevent secondary infections in surgical wounds caused by *Staphylococcus* spp. and/or *Escherichia coli* in dogs (Rosin, 1993). From these data it seems fair to say that the concentration of β-lactam antibiotics in the skin can be, at least, the same as that observed in plasma (Fig. 6).

It should be highlighted that there are specific studies about the penetration of fluoroquinolones in the skin. Several authors have reported that these drugs concentrate in the skin (Schneider, 1996; De Manuelle, 1998). In addition, the MIC values of these antibiotics against many bacteria responsible for infections in the skin are usually low (Meunier, 2004). These two facts can explain why it is possible to administer fluoroquinolones with a longer dosing interval (24 hours) than that described for other antibiotics (Horspool, 2004; Bond, 2005).

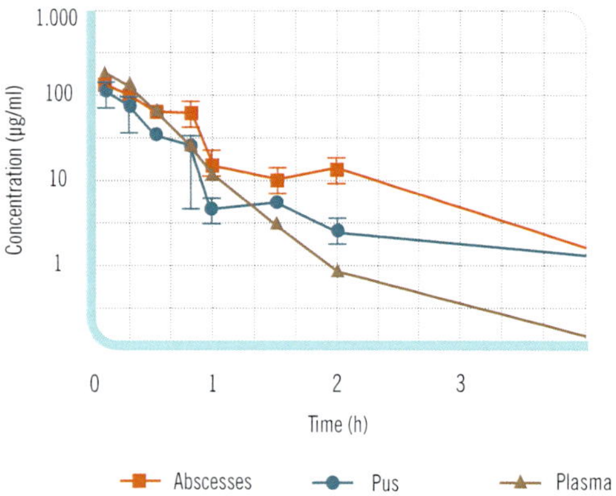

Figure 5. Mean imipenem concentration in plasma (µg/ml), pus (µg/ml) and abscesses (µg/ml) observed after its intravenous administration at a dose of 128 mg/kg live weight/day in an experimental mouse model.

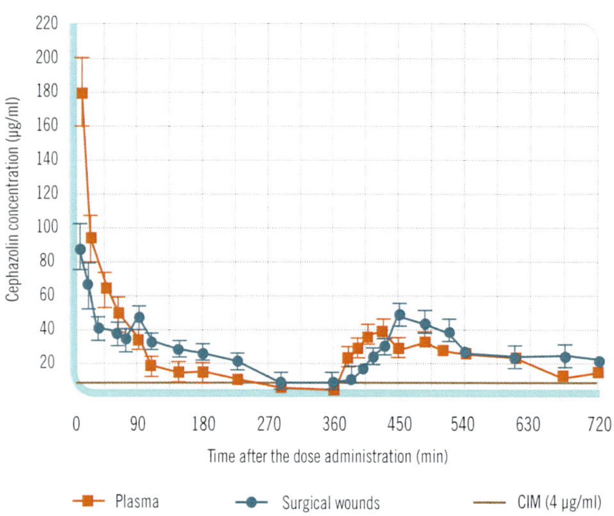

Figure 6. Mean cephazolin concentration in plasma (µg/ml) and surgical wounds (µg/ml) observed after its administration at a dose of 20 mg/kg live weight by intravenous route and at a dose of 20 mg/kg live weight by subcutaneous route 6 hours later in dogs.

Treatment of meningitis

Description of the clinical case in swine

CLINICAL HISTORY

- Farrow-to-finish sow farm of 500 animals.
- Percentage of deaths until the detection of the problem: 1 %.
- The animals had been vaccinated against *Mycoplasma hyopneumoniae* with a commercial vaccine at 7 and 21 days of age.
- An all-in-all-out system by room is used.
- Herd performance before the clinical outbreak: optimum.
- Age of the animals: 5 weeks of age.

CLINICAL SIGNS OBSERVED

- Some animals die suddenly without manifesting any signs.
- The affected animals show signs of ataxia, depression and lack of coordination, followed by lateral recumbency, paddling, convulsions and death (Fig. 7).
- Some are also lame and have swollen joints.
- The mortality rate greatly varies among the different batches, with an average of 9 %
- There are 9 deaths on the day we are notified of the problem.
- There are 10 more animals with this clinical picture on the operation.
- A necropsy of the dead animals is carried out and the following is observed:
    - Cranio-ventral lung consolidation.
- Marked congestion of the brain was observed along with the presence of yellowish fibrinous to fibrino-purulent exudate in the caudoventral area of the cerebellum, and more subtly, on the brain surface (Figs. 8 and 9).

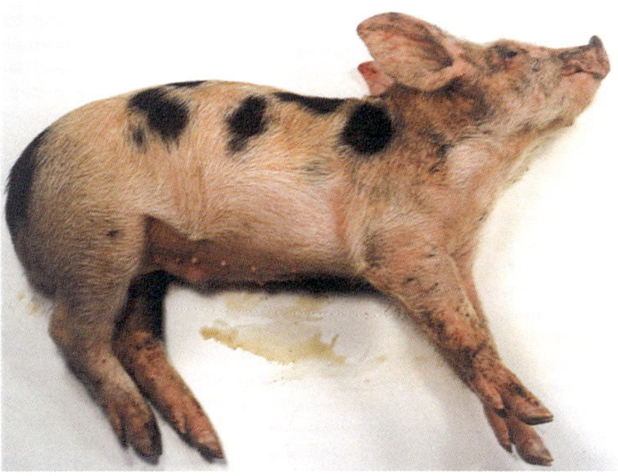

Figure 7

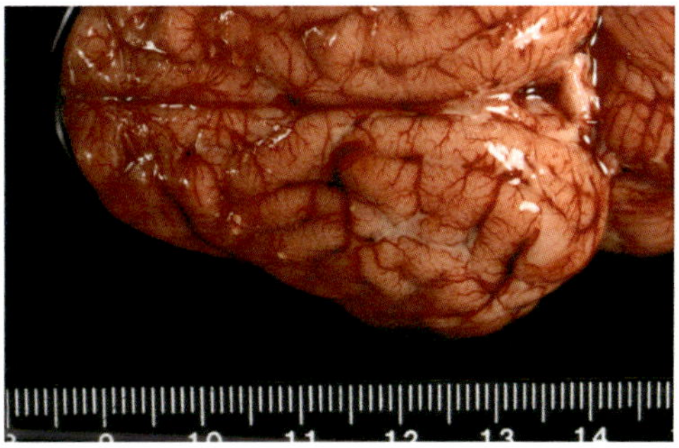

Figure 8

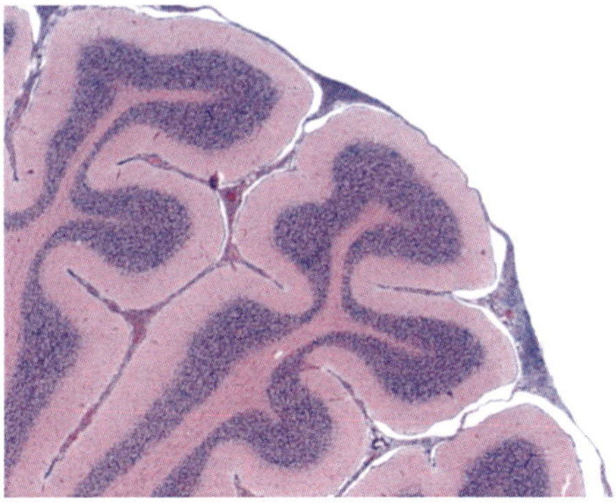

Figure 9

Presumptive diagnosis

- Acute outbreak of streptococcal meningitis.
- The question we should ask ourselves is: Is there a recirculation of the PRRS virus at the same time?

Initial treatment

SYMPTOMATIC

- Dexamethasone at 0.8 mg of active ingredient/kg live weight/day by intramuscular route in a single dose.

AETIOLOGIC

- An antibiotic should be administered to control this bacterial infection. This point will be studied in depth further on.

Brief description of streptococcal meningitis

During the phase of pig production that takes place from 3–4 weeks (piglet weaning) to 7–8 weeks of age (end of transition), clinical problems of meningitis, septicaemia, polyarthritis and other diseases whose responsible aetiological agents are mainly *Streptococcus suis* and *Haemophilus parasuis* very frequently appear (Fig. 10). These diseases imply an increase in the mortality rate and a decrease in the herd's performance that significantly increases the final production cost of fattening pigs.

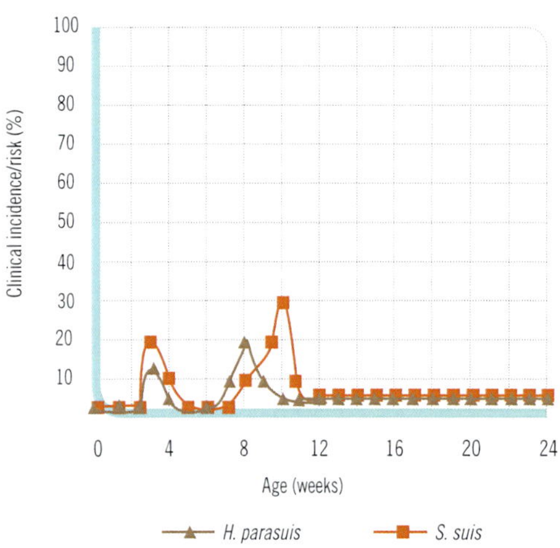

Figure 10. *Streptococcus suis* and *Haemophilus parasuis* epidemiology in pigs (Aarestup et al., 2008)

Streptococcus suis is an early coloniser of the upper airways and genital tract of pigs. They can get infected at birth (in the birth canal) or by direct contact with the mother and other piglets of the litter. *Streptococcus suis (S. suis)* is a major swine pathogen responsible for important economic losses in the swine industry worldwide. It causes a wide variety of diseases in pigs, including meningitis, septicaemia and endocarditis (Gottschalk, 2011). Among the 35 serotypes based on capsular antigens that have been described, serotype 2 is the most frequently isolated from diseased pigs in most countries (Wisselink, 2000). Nowadays, outbreaks of streptococcal infections in pigs are associated with high health farms, farms infected with the PRRS virus and/or operations with a high replacement rate. On the other hand, *S. suis*, especially serotype 2, is also a zoonotic agent. Human cases of *S. suis* infections were first reported in Denmark in 1968 and have been documented in several European and Asian countries as well as in North and South America, Australia and New Zealand. In western countries, *S. suis* infections in humans are most often limited to workers in close contact with pigs or their by-products. However, in Southeast and East Asia, this bacterium also affects the general population and represents a significant public health concern (Gottschalk, 2010).

It is important to highlight that the isolation of *Streptococcus suis* is significant only if this is done out of the upper airways and genital tract of pigs, since they are commensal bacteria in these locations and isolating them there can be considered normal.

CRITICAL REVIEW OF THE TREATMENT

Symptomatic

When there is a bacterial infection in the central nervous system, the bacterial walls of the gram-positive bacteria and the endotoxins released by the gram-negative bacteria stimulate an inflammatory response in the CNS. This inflammatory response activates the complement cascade, prostaglandins and increases the levels of certain cytokines. Morbidity and residual mortality despite the use of bactericidal antibiotics in cases of neonatal bacterial meningitis in children was attributed to this inflammatory response. Therefore, nowadays, the treatment of bacterial meningitis in children focuses on destroying the responsible bacteria by using antibiotics and reducing the harmful effects of the inflammatory response. In animals of veterinary interest, the same approach as with children is used for the treatment of CNS infections. Both glucocorticoids and non-steroidal anti-inflammatory drugs were used to reduce inflammation (Dowling, 1999).

In this case, a single dose of 0.8 mg of dexamethasone/kg live weight/day was administered by intramuscular route. This drug belongs to the glucocorticoid family. These substances are used for the treatment of diseases of the central nervous system because they stabilise microvascular permeability, reduce oedema formation as well as the intracranial pressure and the concentration of free radicals derived from oxygen. The safety and efficacy of glucocorticoids in the treatment of inflammation of the nervous system is not precisely known. In fact, its use and dosage is a topic of debate among internal medicine specialists. It is therefore not surprising that some authors consider that glucocorticoids are contra-indicated in the treatment of bacterial infections of the CNS. However, it is now believed that those drugs are indicated in the treatment of these infections because they reduce the intracranial pressure, brain oedema and the concentration of cytokines in the cerebrospinal fluid. The Academy of American Pediatrics has accepted the use of glucocorticoids and antibiotics for the treatment of bacterial meningitis in children (Dowling, 1999).

Aetiologic

CRITICAL REVIEW OF THE APPLICATION OF ANTIBIOTICS IN THE TREATMENT

Need to use antimicrobials

There is a generalised consensus in the consulted literature about the need to use antibiotics when designing a treatment in clinical cases of bacterial meningitis (Dowling, 1999; Prescott, 2000). It is possible to use antibiotics that belong to the families of quinolones (enrofloxacin, marbofloxacin and danofloxacin), β-lactamics (amoxicillin and cephalosporins), sulfamides and even phenicols (florfenicol).

Therapeutic approach

The elements that should be taken into account are the following:

1. The infection is located in the CNS. More specifically, the affected animals suffer from purulent meningoencephalitis, and the aetiological agent is *Streptococcus suis*.
2. The selected dosage regimen must reach sufficient concentrations at the site of action so they can inhibit bacterial growth and be maintained for a sufficient period of time. In this case, the site of action will be the CNS and the cerebrospinal fluid.
3. The antimicrobial must exert a very fast action since the disease evolves very quickly.

An antibiotic should be chosen taking into account these considerations. In this case, the antimicrobial must be active against *Streptococcus suis*. As explained in the first chapter, antimicrobial susceptibility against *Streptococcus suis* is usually measured with the MIC value. The MIC values of a list of antimicrobials belonging to a wide range of families against *Streptococcus suis* can be seen in Table 2.

The second element that needs to be known is the concentration of the antimicrobial that will be reached at the site of action. Table 1 shows the penetration of several antimicrobials that may be used to treat a *Streptococcus suis* infection in the CNS.

The PK/PD parameters of the antimicrobials that may be used should be calculated for each clinical case in order to predict clinical efficacy in a case by case situation. The different PK/PD parameters calculated for two time-dependent antibiotics, one administered by parenteral route (ceftiofur) and the other usually administered by oral one (amoxicillin), are analysed next as examples.

CEFTIOFUR USE

The first question that needs to be answered is in what animals the administration of cefiofur by parenteral route is indicated. Obviously, all the animals showing clinical signs compatible with streptococcal meningitis should be treated. In addition, given the short period of incubation of this disease as well as the high mortality of the affected animals, antibiotics should be administered to all the animals in the pens where there have been deaths, although these animals are clinically normal. From a strictly pharmacological point of view, it may not seem justified, however, it must be done taking into account the epidemiology and morbidity/mortality of this disease.

In theory, any drug should be administered by intravenous route in the animals that are clinically affected of meningitis to reach maximum plasma concentrations and provide a very high concentration gradient that can really facilitate the passage of the antibiotic to the CNS. However, under practical conditions, this is not a usual route of administration in pigs. In addition, it is recommended to administer antibiotics from 10 to 14 consecutive days in cases of meningitis (in horses for example) depending on the clinical evolution of the disease. Fortunately, there is a commercial presentation that allows ceftiofur concentrations in plasma to be maintained for many days (Fig. 11). Another point that will be revised later on is how to integrate the drug concentration in plasma and in the CNS with the clinical efficacy to treat meningitis in pigs with this drug.

It must be highlighted that many drugs to treat meningitis in pigs by parenteral route (amoxicillin, for example) are usually administered for only 4 consecutive days as a 14-day treatment with a presentation that requires a daily administration would not be realistic. The usual

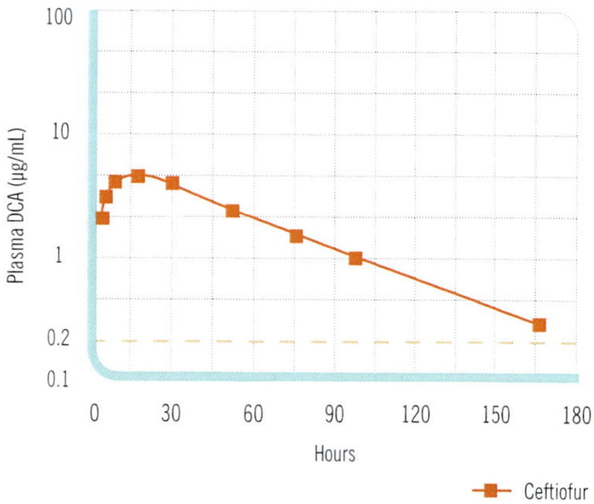

Figure 11. Plasma ceftiofur concentration after the administration of ceftiofur crystalline free acid (ccfa) by intramuscular route in pigs.

treatment (4 or 5 days long) is too short in animals that are clinically affected by meningitis. As a consequence, despite administering this antibiotic treatment, the complete recovery of the clinically affected animals is not very frequent and it is common for the animals to die or suffer from sequelae such as deafness, blindness or purulent arthritis (Sttats, 1997). This is why the administration of amoxicillin by oral route (water and feed) to all the animals that are likely to suffer from this disease is usually carried out. This therapeutic measure is known to significantly reduce the incidence of this disease in the affected herds, although it does not eliminate the status of "carrier" in some animals (Sttats, 1997).

AMOXICILLIN USE

Another possible therapeutic measure consists in the administration of amoxicillin in feed and/or water to the whole population when the disease begins to appear, with the aim of reducing the associated morbidity and mortality (metaphylactic treatment).

The first element that we must know is the concentration of antibiotic that is going to be reached at the site of action. In this case, the site of action for most animals is not the CNS, but the different places where the infection can be controlled before reaching the CNS. As can be observed in Figure 12, it is possible to "block" the infection caused by *Streptococcus suis* before the passage of the germ from the respiratory tract to the bloodstream. It can also be blocked in the blood (septicaemic phase) before it passes to the CNS. Therefore, it is necessary to evaluate the concentration of amoxicillin that can be reached at these three "sites of action" after the administration of this drug according to a standard dosage regimen (20 mg/kg body weight/day).

The most convenient route of administration for this substance in large animal populations is the oral route, mixed with the feed, since it greatly facilitates its administration. It is actually the route of administration most commonly used by swine practitioners when amoxicillin is used as the drug of choice to control clinical cases due to *Streptococcus suis* infection in swine.

In a dosage regimen that involves multiple doses, the total amount of drug administered the first time is not eliminated when the animal ingests the second dose, so that the plasma concentration will be higher after the second dose (principle of superposition). After the administration of several doses, the plasma concentration progressively increases until it reaches a plateau (steady state situation, Figs. 13 and 14). In this situation, the amount of drug administered compensates for the amount eliminated during the dosing interval. The steady state (Css) is reached when 3 or 5 half-lives have gone by (Toutain, 2004). When an antibiotic is administered in feed, the plasma concentration varies throughout the day (from Cmin to Cmax) which perfectly reflects the animals' feeding pattern when the steady state has been reached. Table 3 shows the concentration of amoxicillin that is reached at these three "sites of action" after the administration of this drug by oral route according to a standard dosage regimen.

As we can see, there are no experimental data available about amoxicillin concentrations in the CNS; it is therefore impossible to accurately determine the efficacy of these treatments. However, it can be estimated that the concentration of amoxicillin in the CNS is equal to or higher than 50 % of the concentration in plasma in clinical cases of meningoencephalitis.

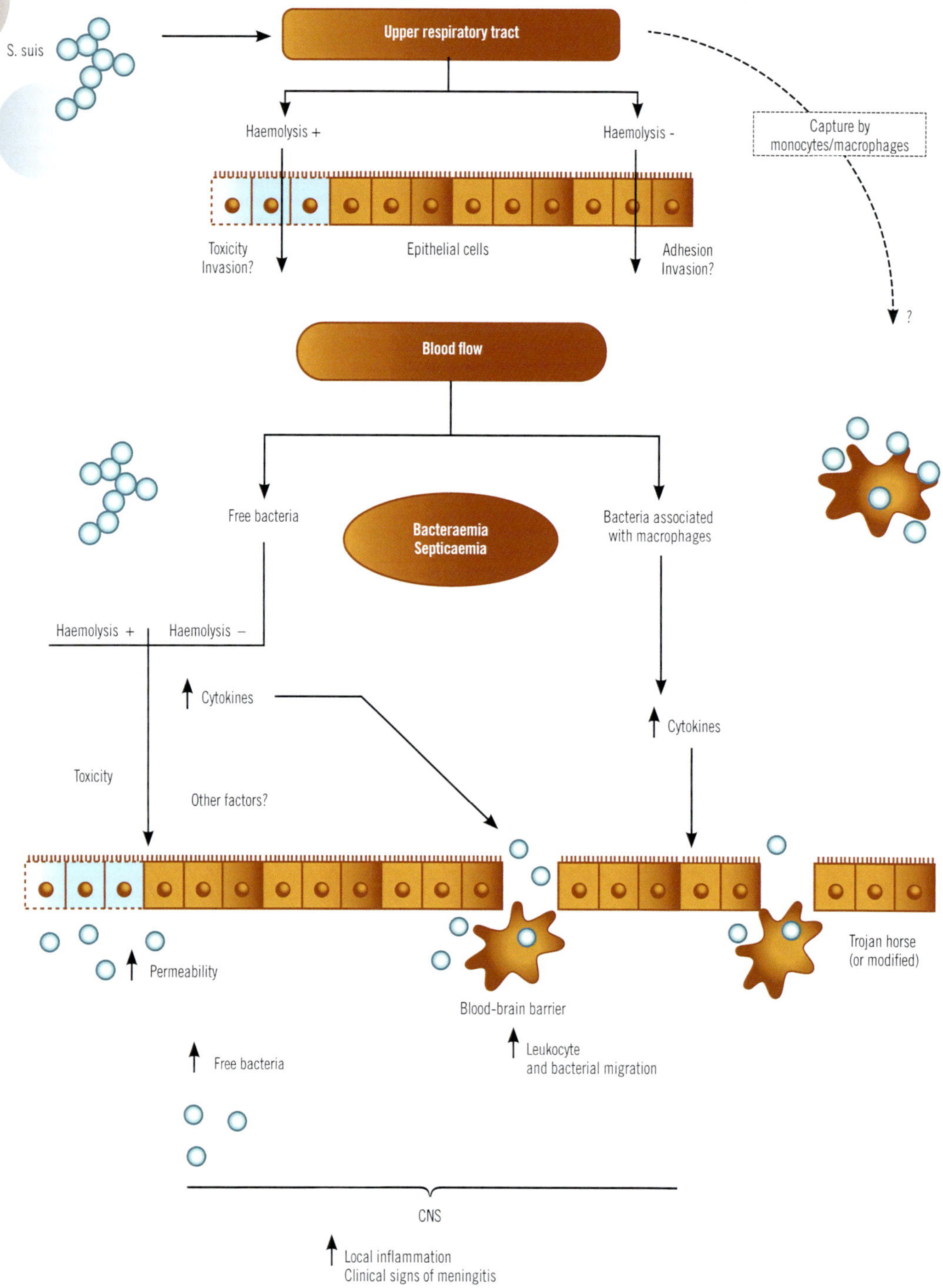

Figure 12. Hypothesis considered to explain the aetiopathogenesis of bacterial meningitis caused by *Streptococcus suis* and sites where it is possible to block the infection by this agent.

A critical point is the selection of the most appropriate antimicrobial treatment depending on the therapeutic objective we want to reach. This objective may vary from the control of the clinical signs to the eradication of the disease. Usually, in the case of streptococcal meningitis in pigs, the therapeutic approach only aims at being effective from a clinical point of view (remission of the signs, improvement of herd performance, etc.). However, it could be interesting to eradicate the microorganism from the affected animals in order to prevent recurrences and/or obtain populations of pigs free from *Streptococcus suis* (Jacobs, 2003; Song 2003). Unfortunately, there is no information available about the PK/PD parameter values for ceftiofur or amoxicillin that can be associated with the eradication of *Streptococcus suis* in infected pigs.

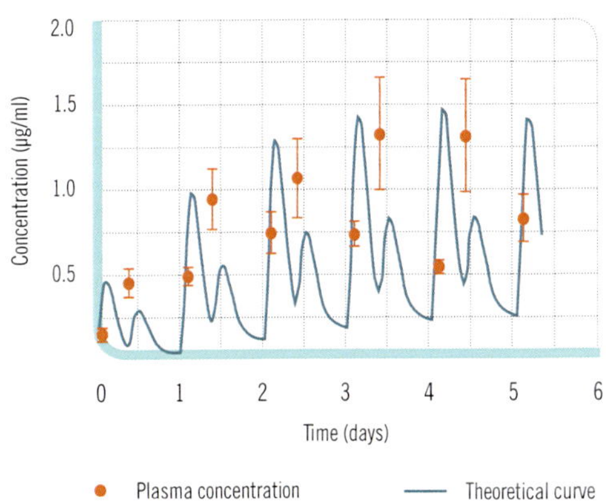

Figure 13. Mean plasma concentration of amoxicillin obtained after the administration to 10 pigs of a commercial presentation in the drinking water.

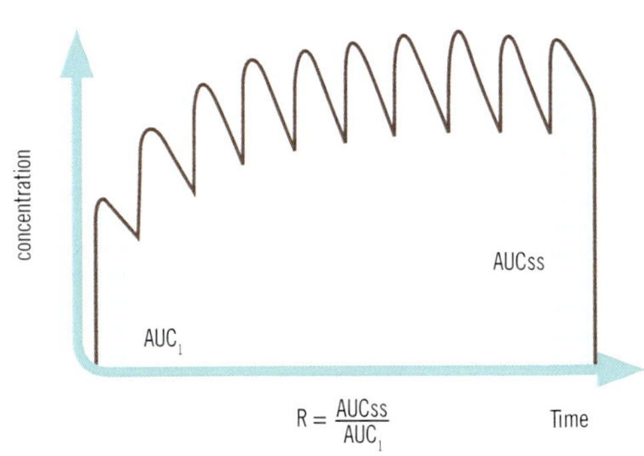

Figure 14

AUC: area under the curve after administration of the first oral dose.
AUCss: area under the curve after reaching the steady state.
R: index of accumulation = AUCss/AUC ratio.

Ceftiofur and amoxicillin are β-lactam antibiotics. Thus, T > MIC is the PK/PD index that best correlates with efficacy. However, in recent studies (McKellar, 2004; McKinnon, 2004), it has been demonstrated that the concentration obtained at steady state (Css) after administering the treatment is key when trying to reduce the pressure of selection of bacterial strains that are resistant in the population. The most appropriate dosage regimen will be that which maintains a Css above the MIC for most of the dosing interval (obviously, it is better if it is maintained for the whole dosing interval) but that prevents the appearance of resistant strains in the population. This objective can be reached if the Css is higher than 5 x MIC. These general concepts can be applied to assess efficacy in the bronchial epithelium and in blood (cases of septicaemia) but they cannot be extended to cases of bacterial meningitis since the parameters that best correlate with efficacy are T > MIC and a Css in the CNS 10-30 higher than the MBC (Figs. 15a and 15b). A reasonable explanation for the difference observed between the treatment of septicaemia and meningitis with the same antibiotic may be the absence of an efficient immune response in the CNS due to a deficiency in immunoglobulins, complement and leukocytes in the cerebrospinal fluid and other parts of the CNS. This is the reason why a higher antibiotic concentration (10–30 times higher than MBC versus 1–5 times higher than the MBC for meningitis and septicaemia, respectively) is necessary for a meningitis treatment to be effective in comparison with a treatment in other organs. As explained in the first chapter, the MIC and MBC are very similar for bactericidal antibiotics (such as amoxicillin and ceftiofur). The MIC value thus gives a good approximation of the bactericidal activity of amoxicillin and cefiofur. This parameter will be taken as a reference pharmacodynamic parameter in the PK/PD models for clinical efficacy.

In the specific case that we are evaluating, a concentration of 0.15 and 0.3 µg/ml (5 x MIC) should be reached to control the infection by *Streptococcus suis* and to avoid the appearance of antimicrobial resistance in the blood and bronchial epithelium for ceftiofur and amoxicillin, respectively. However, this concentration should be much higher (0.3–0.9 µg/ml and 0.6–1.8 µg/ml for ceftiofur and amoxicillin, respectively) in the case of infections that are already located in the CNS. Unfortunately, there is no precise information available about the concentration of ceftiofur and amoxicillin that is really reached at the level of the CNS with the treatments administered and in the animals affected with the disease. Finally, as explained in the first chapter, the treatment of a typical infectious process must have a minimum duration of 4 to 5 days so that the therapeutic objective is reached. Cases of bacterial meningitis are considered an exception and that is why longer treatments are recommended (10–14 days). The duration of the treatment by intramuscular route (4 to 5 days) is usually insufficient to treat infections that are already located in the CNS. However, combination with treatments through drinking water and feed (ideally, both treatments would overlap a little) can be sufficient to address both metaphylaxis and the treatment of clinical cases of streptococcal meningitis in pigs.

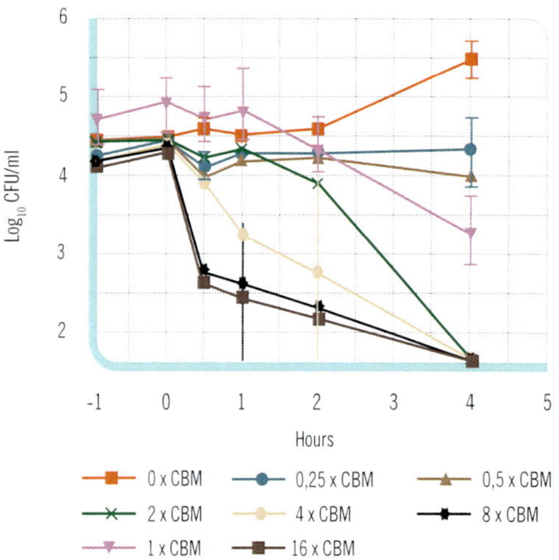

Figure 15a. Mortality curves of *S. pneumoniae* exposed to increasing doses of ceftrioxone.

CFU: Colony forming units.

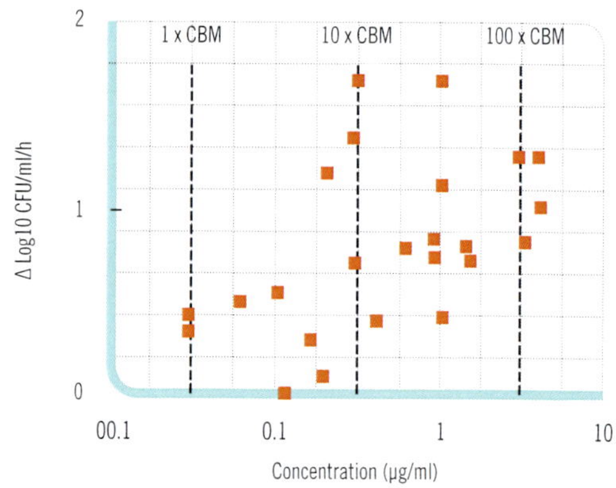

Figure 15b. Bactericidal activity of ceftrioxone in cerebrospinal fluid.

CFU: Colony forming units.

Finally, the likelihood of clinical success for the antimicrobials that may be used for the treatment of *Streptococcus suis* infections can be calculated taking into account the pharmacokinetic and pharmacodynamic information provided by the pharmaceutical companies or available in the literature (Table 4). Nevertheless, the likelihood of success will depend on the target tissue (CNS or other tissues).

The information provided in Table 4 is for guidance only since each particular strain has its own MIC value for each antimicrobial. The PK/PD parameters of the antimicrobials that may be used should therefore be calculated for each clinical case and the result should be taken into account to optimise the therapy and choose the best antimicrobial option (see Fig. 14 in chapter 2). In addition, in order to choose an appropriate antimicrobial agent, swine practitioners should know the efficacy of the molecule (previously analysed), the current regulations on the use of antimicrobials in their country and the history of the herd.

Treatment of skin infections

Description of the clinical case in swine

CLINICAL HISTORY

- Farrow-to-finish sow farm of 800 animals.
- Percentage of dead pigs until the detection of the problem: 2 %.
- The animals had been vaccinated against *Mycoplasma hyopneumoniae* at 7 and 21 days of age with a commercial vaccine.
- An all-in-all-out system by room is used.
- Herd performance before the clinical outbreak: optimum.
- Age of the animals: 7 weeks of age

CLINICAL SIGNS OBSERVED

- The affected animals show signs of depression.
- Their skin becomes reddish and then coppery, thin scales are observed in the intertrigenous areas of the axillae and groin and other parts of the body. (Figs. 16 and 17).
- Lesions progress to cover the whole body with a greasy brown exudate.
- The mortality rate greatly varies among the different batches, with an average of 8 %.
- There are 2 deaths on the day we are notified of the problem; the dead pigs show clear signs of cachexia.
- There are 50 more animals with this clinical picture on the farm.

A necropsy of the dead animals is carried out and the following is observed:

- Cranio-ventral lung consolidation.
- The histopathological findings include an intraepidermal subcorneal vesicular and pustular dermatitis, together with neutrophils, bacteria and acantholytic keratinocytes (Figs. 18 and 19).

Presumptive diagnosis

- Acute outbreak of exudative epidermitis.
- The question we should ask ourselves is: Is there a recirculation of the PRRS virus at the same time?

Initial treatment

AETIOLOGIC

- An antibiotic should be administered to control this bacterial infection. This point will be analysed in depth further on.

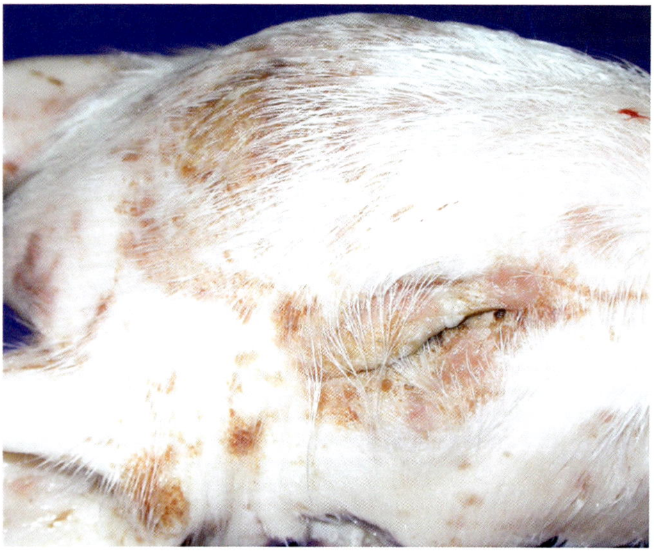

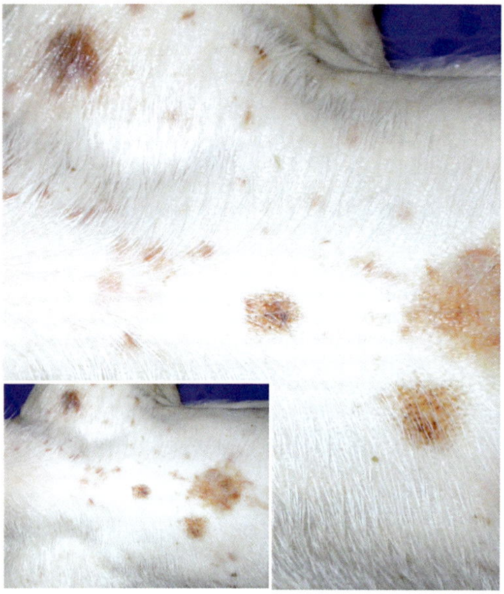

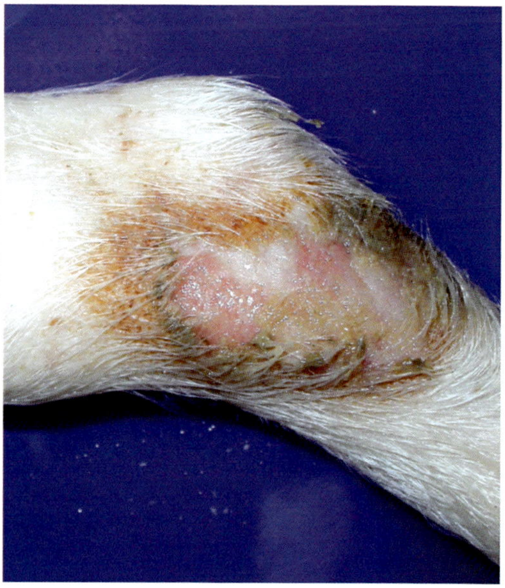

Figures 16 and 17. Pig with exudative epidermitis.

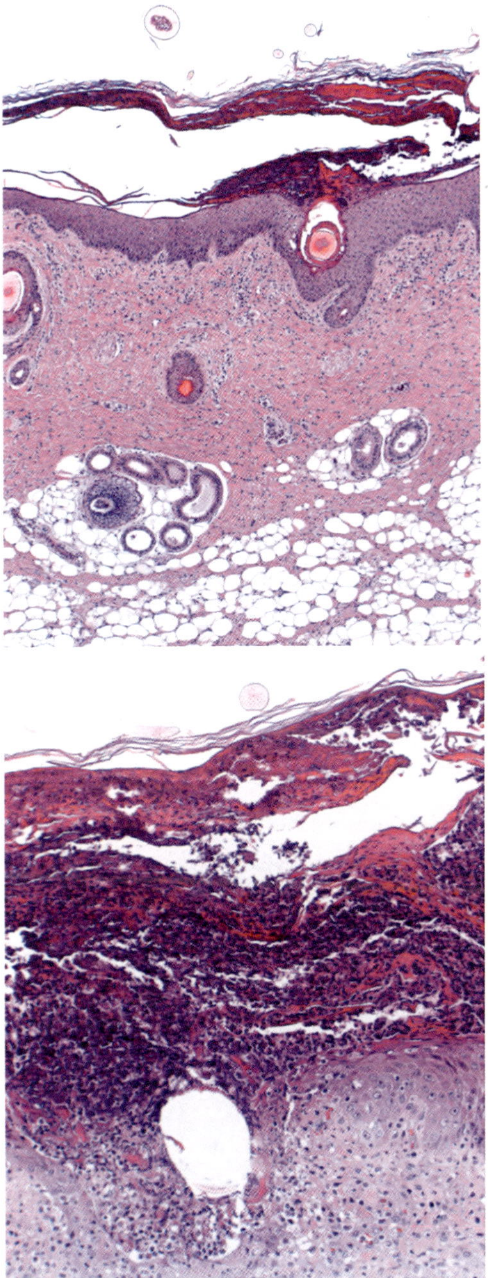

Figures 18 and 19. Hispopathological lesion observed in pigs with exudative epidermitis.

BRIEF DESCRIPTION OF EXUDATIVE EPIDERMITIS

Greasy pig disease or exudative epidermitis (EE) is a readily and widely recognised condition of pigs, especially piglets and weaners, that is sporadically reported to cause significant morbidity and mortality in naive herds (Allaker, 1990; Wegener, 2006). The main cause of EE is thought to be pathogenic strains of *Staphylococcus hyicus* (*S. hyicus*) harbouring toxins. It is assumed that piglets are exposed to bacteria at birth as they pass through the vagina; consequently, *S. hyicus* can be isolated from the skin of newborn piglets (Allaker, 1990). For infection to become established and disease to develop, it is assumed that this commensal organism, which is carried by pigs (on the conjunctiva, snout and ear skin and vagina) and may also survive in the environment, must gain entry via skin abrasions such as those that may occur due to fights between piglets, unclipped teeth or rough floor or wall conditions (Taylor, 2006). The presence of the porcine circovirus type 2 and porcine parvovirus has been suggested as a predisposing factor, although such viruses are concurrent and common factors in commercial pig herds (Kim, 2004). A key feature of the pathogenesis of this skin disease is the presence of bacterial strains that express exfoliative toxins known as ExhA, ExhB, ExhC, ExhD, SHETA and SHETB. The Exh toxins have been shown to digest desmoglein-1 in the epidermis of pig skin. Consequently, this disease process is considered to involve the same mechanisms as staphylococcal scalded skin syndrome and bullous impetigo in humans (Nihisifuji, 2008; Olivry, 2009). There may be other staphylococcal species involved, and an exfoliative toxin similar to ExhB has been isolated from *S. chromogenes* isolated from healthy pigs. Experimental infection of pigs with this isolate led to clinical signs of EE (Andresen, 2005). Naturally occurring cases of EE with

S. chromogenes were reported by the Animal Health and Veterinary Laboratories Agency (AHVLA) in 2005. An exfoliative toxin gene similar to ExhC was isolated from a field isolate of *Staphylococcus sciuri* that was associated with field infection and EE in piglets from a breeding herd; EE was experimentally reproduced in piglets by feeding or injecting the bacterial isolate, which led to a fatal outcome (Chen, 2007).

A variable number of piglets may be affected within a litter and clinical signs may be observed from 4 days of age to 6 weeks old. Skin lesions may vary in terms of their distribution and severity. The skin becomes reddish and then coppery, and thin scales develop in the intertrigenous areas of the axillae and groin; lesions may progress to cover the whole body with a greasy brown exudate. Ulcers may be observed in the mouth, and there may be erosions of the coronary band and heel areas. A skin lesion consisting of vesicles/pustules involving the nose, lips, tongue and coronary band may be seen in the peracute form of the disease. Piglets die from anorexia and dehydration, and others will be stunted and have localised lesions with a yellow-brown skin and flaking in the axillae, groin, carpal joints and face. In early lesions in the abdominal area, gentle pressure and traction can peel the skin. In adult pigs, brown skin lesions may be observed on the back or flanks. Infection of piglets with *S. hyicus* can also be associated with septic arthritis in the absence of skin lesion (Wegener, 2006; Allaker, 1990). The diagnosis of EE is fairly straightforward with the disease is severe and generalised. It can be confirmed by collecting samples for bacterial culture and skin biopsies. The histopathological findings typically include an intraepidermal, subcorneal, vesicular and pustular dermatitis, with neutrophils, bacteria and acantholytic keratinocytes. Other common histopathological changes include acanthosis, crusting, exfoliation and exocytosis (Olivry, 2009; Nishifuji, 2008). The diseases that may be considered in the differential diagnosis include swine pox, sarcoptic mange, dermatophytosis, pityriasis rosea, zinc deficiency, biotin deficiency, dermatosis vegetans of Landrace pigs, and traumatic wounds due to abrasions or fighting. In rare situations associated with exotic or notifiable disease outbreaks, it may also be possible to see lesions that arise from viral infections associated with vesicular diseases (foot and mouth, swine vesicular disease, vesicular stomatitis and vesicular exanthema). A dual infection with *S. hyicus* and *Dermatophilus congolensis is possible* (Lomax, 1983). Pustular dermatitis may also be seen in piglets associated with streptococcal infection (Cameron, 2006).

Management of EE can be challenging when an outbreak develops in a naive herd, and it is assumed that there is some form of acquired immunity; consequently, autogenous vaccines have sometimes been used. Prevention is obviously better than treatment since piglet mortality can be high. The hygiene and management of the facilities where the piglets are housed should be carefully examined to include meticulous washing and disinfection of the unit and of sows entering the farrowing unit. Piglets with skin lesions can be treated topically and systemically. Antibacterial resistance patterns for *S. hyicus* isolates may reflect the local use of antimicrobial agents for controlling other diseases associated with the respiratory or gastrointestinal tract. Such resistance patterns can be difficult to predict, and it is important to analyse the herd's history, including previous antimicrobial use, when choosing an antibacterial treatment. Given that not all cases of EE are due to *S. hyicus*, it is important to have bacterial culture and sensitivity testing carried out when treating large numbers of pigs (Taylor, 2006; Burch, 2008).

CRITICAL REVIEW OF THE TREATMENT

SYMPTOMATIC

In principle, no symptomatic treatment was administered in this clinical case but it may be advisable to administer fluids to the affected piglets.

AETIOLOGIC

In this case, the aetiological treatment focuses on controlling the infection caused by *Staphylococcus hyicus* using antibiotics.

CRITICAL REVIEW OF THE ADMINISTRATION OF ANTIBIOTICS IN THE TREATMENT

Need to use antibiotics

There is a wide consensus among swine practitioners about the need to use antimicrobials in cases of exudative epidermitis (Prescott, 2000). It is possible to use antibiotics that belong to the families of cephalosporins, other β-lactams (e.g. amoxicillin-clavulanic acid) and even quinolones (enrofloxacin and marbofloxacin). These antibiotics are also used to treat canine pyoderma caused by *Staphylococcus intermedius* (Ganiere, 2001; Bloom, 2001; Muller, 2001).

Therapeutic approach

The elements that should be taken into account are the following:

1. The infection is located in the skin.
2. The chosen dosage regimen must allow sufficient concentrations to be reached at the site of action so they can inhibit the growth of the bacteria and be maintained for a sufficient period of time. Ideally, the drug should concentrate in the skin.

Treatment with an antimicrobial will be effective in this case if the necessary concentration of the product is reached in the skin. As a general concept, it can be said that the treatment of a typical infectious process must last from 3 to 7 days for the therapeutic objective to be reached. However, treatments of skin infections are considered an exception in pets and a 3-week treatment is recommended in cases of superficial canine pyoderma and a 4-week treatment is recommended for deep canine pyoderma. In addition, it is considered essential to continue the treatment for 10 and 14 more days after the remission of the clinical signs for superficial and deep pyoderma, respectively, in order to avoid the appearance of recurrences, which are usually very frequent in this disease (Bond, 2005). In any case, the duration of the treatment must be adapted to each case since there are great individual variations in the response. In the case of the treatment of exudative epidermitis in pigs, a 5-day treatment may be enough if the animals are treated at the very beginning of the infectious process (Fraile, personal communication). However, a treatment duration much closer to that recommended for pets (2-3 weeks) may be necessary in animals that are treated when the infectious process is well established in the animal.

An antibiotic should be chosen taking into account these considerations. In this case, the first point to be analysed is that the antimicrobial must be active against *Staphylococcus hyicus*. As seen in the first chapter, antimicrobial susceptibility is usually measured with the MIC value. The MIC values of a list of antimicrobials that may be used in a *Staphylococcus hyicus* infection are listed in Table 5.

The MIC for amoxicillin and *Staphylococcus hyicus* is 8 μg/ml. However, the MIC value for amoxicillin and this bacterium is 0.5 μg/ml when amoxicillin and clavulanic acid are jointly administered.

The second element that needs to be known is the concentration of the antimicrobial that will be reached at the site of action. In this case, the site of action is the skin. Table 6 shows the penetration after parenteral administration of the antimicrobials that may be used to treat a *Staphylococcus hyicus* infection in this location.

The PK/PD parameters of the antimicrobials that may be used should be calculated for each clinical case in order to predict clinical efficacy in a case by case situation. The different PK/PD parameters calculated for a one time-dependent antibiotic (amoxicillin- clavulanic acid) are analysed next as examples.

Amoxicillin and clavulanic acid are β-lactam antibiotics. The first drug is a well-known antibiotic of this family and clavulanic acid, produced by *Streptomyces clavuligenus*, has a chemical structure similar to some β-lactamines, e.g. penicillin. When clavulanic acid is present in the extra-cellular space of bacteria it competitively binds and inactivates β-lactamases. These enzymes (β-lactamases) are produced by bacteria and found in their extracellular space (gram-positive bacteria) or peri-plasmatic space (gram-negative bacteria). When β-lactamases interact with β-lactamines, they bind to each other. The binding causes the opening of the structure of β-lactamines and the loss of their bactericidal activity, as illustrated in Figure 20a. How clavulanic acid exerts its function (Fig. 20b) is also represented.

As explained in previous chapters, the T > MIC (time of the dosing interval during which the plasma concentration is above the MIC) is the PK/PD parameter that best correlates with efficacy for these antibiotics. Thus, the most appropriate dosage regimen will be that which can maintain a Css (steady-state concentration) above the MIC for most of the dosing interval (obviously, it is better if it is maintained during the whole dosing interval). Experimental and clinical studies have determined that this PK/PD parameter (T > MIC) must reach a value close to 50 % of the dose interval to achieve optimum

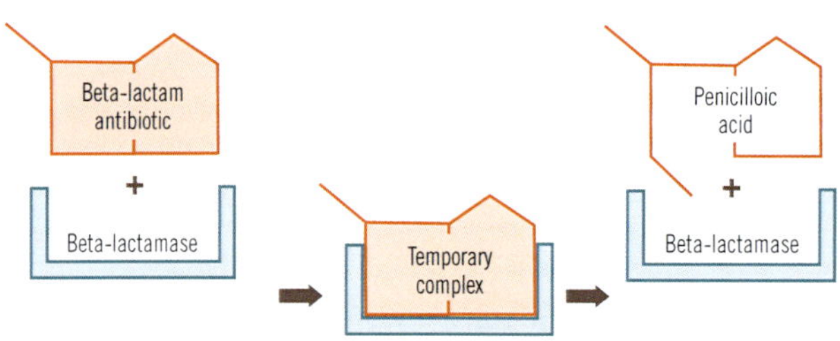

Figure 20a. Mechanism of action of β-lactamase enzymes.

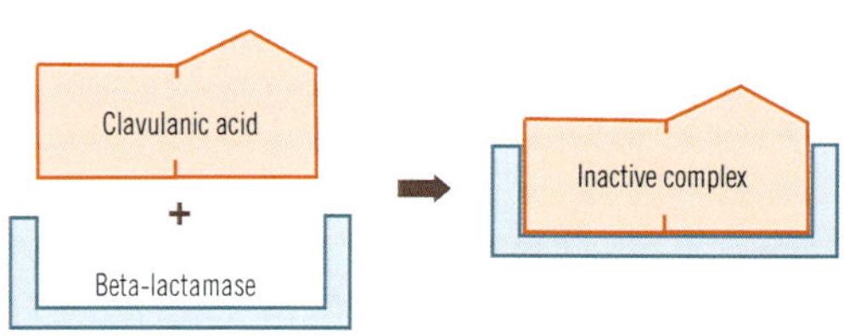

Figure 20b. Mechanism of action of clavulanic acid.

clinical efficacy and/or bacteriological cure in the case of β-lactam antibiotics (Adamson, 1985; Craig, 2004; McKellar, 2004). It would be ideal to know this information in the case of the treatment of skin infections. Unfortunately, the author has not found any data and we will therefore assume that these same parameters can be extrapolated in the case of the treatment of these infections. In conclusion, the objective will be to obtain a steady state concentration (Css) of 0.5 µg/ml (1 x MIC) and a T > MIC of at least 50 % of the dose interval after administering amoxicillin and clavulanic acid by intramuscular route for the treatment to be effective (McKellar, 2004; Ganiere, 2005).

Unfortunately, it was not possible to find public information about the pharmacokinetics of amoxicillin and clavulanic acid in pigs. However, it was possible to find the plasma concentration of both drugs after the administration in very young calves (less than one week old) of 7 mg/kg body weight/day of amoxicillin and 1,75 mg/kg body weight/day of clavulanic acid. We can thus analyse if this pharmacokinetic profile is close to that observed in pigs. On the one hand, amoxicillin is essentially cleared through the kidney. It would therefore not be necessary to make any type of adjustment for the dose in young pigs since the essential pharmacokinetic parameters (plasma clearance) that determine the dosage regimen remain constant during the development of the animal. However, these basic parameters could be modified for other antibiotics in young individuals of other species and this should be taken into account when establishing a dosage regimen. Pigs are born with well-developed kidneys; the dosage regimen during development should therefore not be modified in relation to that of adults if the drug studied is essentially cleared through this organ. Short and Clarke (1984) point out, referring to penicillins, that their dosage does not require any type of adjustment from the second or third day of life also in neonate calves. All these data suggest that the pharmacokinetic profile for both drugs is very similar in young calves and pigs.

The repeated administration of multiple doses of a drug at regular intervals that are shorter than 5 half-lives leads to the accumulation of the drug until it reaches steady state. This state of "equilibrium" is reached when 3 to 5 half-lives have gone by (Baggot, 2001). In this specific case, both drugs are administered with a dosing interval of 24 hours. After the first administration, in this specific case, the total amount of administered drug is almost completely eliminated when the animal receives the second dose so there is no phenomenon of accumulation of the drug until steady state is reached (Fig. 21). In this specific case, the dosing interval is 24 hours. The T > MIC parameter thus has a value close to 100 % of the dose interval. It should be highlighted that the concentration of amoxicillin is observed in plasma and the site of action is the skin; however, as explained previously, the concentration in the skin can be, at least, the same as the one observed in plasma.

Finally, the probability of clinical success for the antimicrobials that may be used for the treatment of *Staphylococcus hyicus* infections can be calculated taking into account the pharmacokinetic and pharmacodynamic information provided by the pharmaceutical companies or available in the literature (Table 7).

The information provided in Table 7 is for guidance only since each particular strain has its own MIC value for each antimicrobial. The PK/PD parameters of the antimicrobials that may be used should therefore be calculated for each clinical case and the result should be taken into account to optimise the therapy and choose the best antimicrobial option (see

Fig. 14 in chapter 2). In addition, in order to choose an appropriate antimicrobial agent, swine practitioners should know the efficacy of the molecule (previously analysed), the current regulations on the use of antimicrobials in their country and the history of the herd.

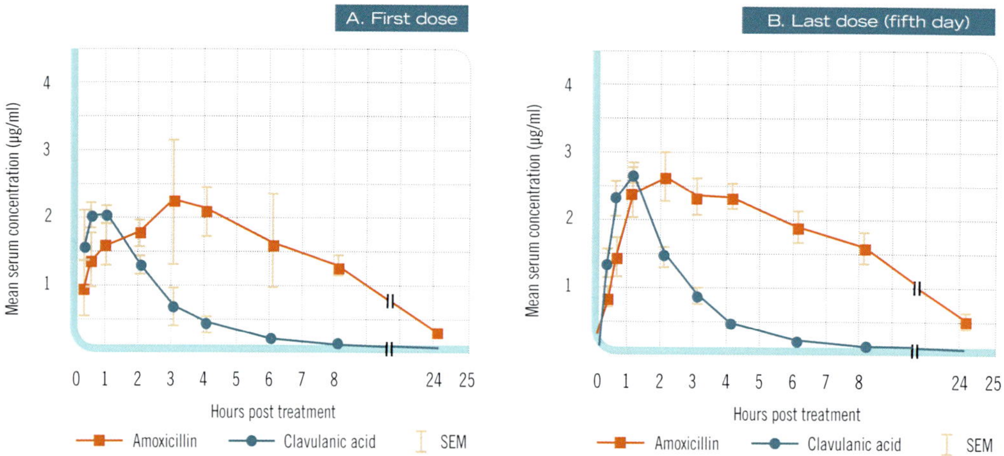

Figure 21. Amoxicillin and clavulanic acid serum concentration after the administration of an intramuscular dose of 7 mg/kg b.w./day of amoxicillin and 1.75 mg/kg b.w./day of clavulanic acid in neonate calves for five days.

Table 1. Penetration of antimicrobials in the CNS.

High penetration	Low penetration
Fluoroquinolones	Penicillins*
Doxycycline	Cephalosporins*
Phenicols	Aminoglycosides
Sulphonamides	Tetracyclines
	Macrolides

*Higher penetration in inflamed tissues.

Table 2. MIC of antimicrobials for the treatment of a *Streptococcus suis* infection (Wisselink, 2006 and author's data).

Antimicrobial	MIC range (μg/ml)	MIC_{90} (μg/ml)
Ceftiofur	0.03-0.13	0.03
Enrofloxacin	0.06-1	0.5
Florfenicol	0.5-4	2
Gentamicin	0.5-16	8
Penicillin	0.13-2	0.13
Amoxicillin	0.03-1	0.06
Tetracycline	0.13- > 128	64
Tilmicosin	0.13-128	128
Spectinomycin	2-128	16
Trimethroprim/Sulfamethoxazole	0.06-16	2

Table 3. Amoxicillin concentration in the bronchial epithelium, blood and CNS after the administration of a standard dosage regimen (20 mg/kg body weight/day) in pigs.

Concentration	Bronchial epithelium*	Blood	CNS**
Minimum	0.172	0.52	0.26
Maximum	0.541	1.64	0.82
Average	0.356	1.08	0.54

* Data estimated from scientific publications (Agerso, 1998).

** Data estimated from scientific publications about other related drugs (we assume that the concentration in the CNS is 50 % of the concentration in plasma).

Table 4. Probability of clinical success for antimicrobials in the treatment of *Streptococcus suis* infections.

Antimicrobial group	**Example**	**PK/PD parameter and threshold value**	**Probability of success in CNS (real treatment of meningitis)**	**Probability of success in other tissues (mainly control)**
Fluoroquinolones	Marbofloxacin Danofloxacin Enrofloxacin	AUC/MIC > 100? andT > MIC?$	+/++*	+/++
Cephalosporins	Ceftiofur	T > MIC	++/+++*	+++
ß-lactams (no cephalosporins)	Amoxicillin Penicillin	T > MIC	+/++*	++/+++
Aminoglycosides	Neomycin	Cmax/MIC > 10	-	-
Phenicols	Florfenicol	T > MIC	+/++*&	+/++&
Macrolides	Tilmicosin	T > MIC	-	-

Probability of success: - failure, + low, ++ intermediate and +++ high.
*It depends on the time between the onset of the clinical signs and the treatment. The shorter this time; the better the efficacy of the treatment.
$ There is little information available about the PK/PD parameters that may be correlated with the clinical efficacy of quinolones in the treatment of *Streptococcus suis* infections. A time-dependent activity for gram-positive germs (e.g. *Staphylococci*) has been reported in the case of marbofloxacin.
& No scientific data is available about the use of phenicols to treat *Streptococcus suis* infections. However, there are clinical data that support this information (Fraile, personal communication).

Table 5. MIC of antimicrobials for the treatment of *Staphylococcus hyicus* infection (Wegener, 1994; Futagawa-Saito, 2009).

	Wegener et al., 1994		**Futagawa-Saito, 2009**	
Antimicrobial	**MIC range (μg/ml)**	**MIC_{90} (μg/ml)**	**MIC range (μg/ml)**	**MIC_{90} (μg/ml)**
Enrofloxacin	0.13-0.5	0.25	-	-
Ofloxacin	-	-	0.25-1	-
Ampicillin	< 0.03-2	0.5	0.12- > 16	-
Penicillin	-	-	< 0.06- > 8	
Cephalosporins (cefuroxime)	-	-	< 0.5-2	
Streptomycin	1- > 64	> 64	-	-
Phenicols (chloramphenicol)	-	-	4-64	-

Table 6. Penetration of antimicrobials in the skin.

Antimicrobial group	Example	Penetration at the site of action
Fluoroquinolones	Marbofloxacin Danofloxacin	++/+++
β-lactams	Amoxicillin	++/+++*
Cephalosporins	Ceftiofur	++/+++*

-, no, + low, ++ intermediate and +++ high penetration.

* Penetration in inflamed tissues.

Table 7. Probability of clinical success for antimicrobials in the treatment of *Staphylococcus hyicus* infections.

Antimicrobial group	Example	PK/PD parameter and threshold value	Probability of success
Fluoroquinolones	Marbofloxacin Danofloxacin Enrofloxacin	AUC/MIC > 100? and T > MIC?$	+/++*&
Cephalosporins	Ceftiofur	T > MIC	++/+++*
ß-lactams (no cephalosporins)	Amoxicillin Penicillin	T > MIC	-/+*
Combination of ß-lactams	Amoxicillin Clavulanic acid	T > MIC	++/+++*
Aminoglycosides	Neomycin	Cmax/MIC > 10	-
Fenicols	Florfenicol	T > MIC	-
Macrolides	Tilmicosin	T > MIC	-

Probability of success: - failure, + low, ++ intermediate and +++ high.

*It depends on the time between the onset of the clinical signs and the treatment. The shorter this time; the better the efficacy of the treatment.

$ There is little information about the PK/PD parameter that may be correlated with the clinical efficacy of quinolones in the treatment of *Staphylococcus hyicus* infections. A time-dependent activity for gram-positive germs (e.g. *Staphylococci*) has been reported in the case of marbofloxacin.

& No scientific data is available about the use of quinolones to treat *Staphylococcus hyicus* infections. However, this group of drugs are widely used to treat skin infections due to *Staphylococcus intermedius* in dogs (Fraile, personal communication).

5

Treatment of mastitis metritis agalactia syndrome in sows

Treatment of mastitis metritis agalactia syndrome in sows

5

General concepts

Mastitis metritis agalactia syndrome in sows: a complex syndrome

In their first days of life, piglets are totally reliant on the sow for access to colostrum and milk. In general, more than 50 % of piglet deaths occur in the first 4 days after birth, and piglets are most vulnerable in their first 24 hours of life (Marchant, 2000). Inadequate colostrum intake may cause the death of piglets due to starvation and hypothermia. A low colostrum intake is associated with a low weight gain during first three days postpartum (Milligan, 2002). For this reason, any alteration in both milk yield and composition has a considerable impact on piglet weight gain and growth rate.

Postparturient disorders, including dysgalactia in sows, are a very important disease complex from an economic point of view (Bertschinger, 1999). They are reported worldwide, but subsumed under different terms depending on the geographical location. While mastitis, metritis and agalactia syndrome (MMA) (Martin, 1967) is commonly used in European countries, postpartum dysgalactia syndrome (PPDS or PDS) has become widely accepted in English-speaking areas. Postpartum dysgalactia syndrome (PDS) in sows is characterised by inadequate and insufficient colostrum and milk production during the first days after farrowing (Klopfenstein, 2006). Although PDS is still considered as a major problem in practice, recent scientific information is scarce. Bäckström (1984) found an incidence of MMA of 6.9 % (ranging from 1.1 %-37.2 %) in 16,405 newly-farrowed sows in 31 sow herds in Illinois, USA. In a study which included 27,656 newly-farrowed sows conducted in the area of Missouri, a 13 % incidence of MMA was found (Threlfall, 1973). The incidence of MMA in Swedish herds has been reported to range from 5.5 % in small herds to 10.3 % in large herds (Bäckström, 1973).

A number of postpartum lactation problems are certainly the consequence of some inflammatory process associated with localised or systemic infections. The main clinical signs of a diseased sow in the postpartum period are fever (> 40 °C), lethargy, anorexia and constipation. The main diseases affecting postpartum and lactating sows are urinary tract infections, endometritis and mastitis. Endometritis occurs following parturition as a result of dystocia, traumatic injuries, abortion and unhygienic manipulations. Pyometra, an acute or chronic suppurative inflammation of the uterus with accumulation of large quantities of pus, is rare in sows. The gross and microscopic pathological examination of the reproductive systems of diseased and normal sows in the postpartum period suggests that endometritis is rare (Ringarp, 1960; Jones, 1976; Middleton-Williams, 1977) whereas lactation problems seem to be more frequent in sows with renal infection (Berner, 1984, 1988). Even though metritis is often a part of the syndrome, mastitis is the central symptom, as shown by several studies (Ross, 1981; Heinritzi, 1999). On the other hand, a purulent vulvar discharge with or without blood may be observed in cases of cystitis/pyelonephritis and should be differentiated from that originating from the genital tract. The discharge usually contains mucus, is associated with urination, especially at the end of stream, and is not related to the oestrous cycle. To confirm urinary tract infections, urinalyses should be performed on samples of affected animals or on samples collected at slaughter.

Mastitis is a clear pathological entity: infected glands typically show signs of inflammation such as severe oedema and skin congestion (Klopfenstein, 2006). It can be a local process, restricted to one or several glands, but can also affect many mammary complexes. Moreover, sows develop fever (> 40.3 °C) and lose their appetite (Halgaard, 1983) when many glands are involved. Under normal conditions, milk contains a certain amount of somatic cells per millilitre. The predominant cell types are macrophages (35-79 %), T and B lymphocytes (10-24 %), polymorphonuclear leukocytes (3-26 %) and desquamated epithelial cells (2-15 %). However, the invasion of the mammary gland by microorganisms leads to an increase in the number of somatic cells in the milk and most of those (nearly 100 %) are polymorphonuclear leukocytes as it has been described for cows (Gruet, 2001).

The clinical appearance of MMA in sows is usually diagnosed via rectal temperature (Furniss, 1987) and sows are defined as "PPDS-positive" when a certain threshold is exceeded. This threshold is defined rather coincidentally between 39.3 °C and 40.5 °C and its use might be regarded as critical since physiological hyperthermia is often observed in sows, leading to misinterpretations (Klopfenstein, 2006). To avoid confusion with this physiological temperature increase and to reduce the administration of antibiotics in non-affected animals, a threshold of 39.5 °C in the 12 to 24 hours postpartum is recommended. Furthermore, the diagnosis should be based not only on a high temperature, but also on a combination of appropriate criteria such as clinical changes in the mammary glands, a reduced milk production and a loss of appetite (Larsen, 2006). Other parameters such as the cell count, established for cows' milk, are not commonly used for the diagnosis of this disorder and data on thresholds are rare. For instance, a threshold of 5×10^6 cells per ml was proposed by Bertschinger (1990), while Persson (1996) suggested 10×10^6 cells per mL in sows.

The bacteria most frequently isolated from mastitis-affected sows belong to the class of coliforms (Kemper, 2006). Bacterial genera included in the class of coliforms are represented by *Escherichia*, *Enterobacter*, *Citrobacter*, and *Klebsiella*. Several successful infection experiments leading to mastitis in sows have demonstrated the predominant role of these organisms (Hirsch, 2003) but bacteria of the genera *Staphylococcus* and *Streptococcus* spp. may also be involved. The predominant role of coliform bacteria was clearly shown by Wegmann (1986): in 131 complexes with mastitis, *E. coli* and *Klebsiella pneumoniae* were isolated in 79 % of the cases. This importance of *E. coli* has been confirmed in several studies (Pedersen, 1998; Persson, 1997) and in infection experiments, provoking clinical and haematological changes comparable to natural infections (Ross, 1983). Bacteria causing or at least accompanying coliform mastitis may come from the intestinal flora of the sow, from the environment or from the oral flora of the neonatal piglet. The hypothesis of a galactogenous route of infection was corroborated by experiments in which a reduction of PPDS prevalence could be noticed after protecting the mammary gland against faecal contamination. Therefore, faecal contamination was postulated to be of paramount importance as a cause of puerperal mastitis. The faecal origin of *E. coli* isolated from sows' milk was also reported by Awad Masalmeh (1990): in one quarter of 67 PPDS-affected sows, identical O-serogroup *E. coli* were detected in both milk and faecal samples.

The lack of gram-negative bacteria culture growth in uterine samples supports the theory that uterine involvement in PPDS is of minor importance, as has been suggested in several studies (Armstrong, 1968; Nachreiner, 1974). However, infections of the urinary tract are strongly related to puerperal diseases, even though urinary infections are not apparent clinically (Mauch, 2004). In these infections as well, the most common organism associated with bacteriuria was found to be *E. coli* (Waller, 2002). Therefore, not only faecal, but also urine contamination has to be considered as an a source of infection for PPDS. Bertschinger (1999) suggested that the often recommended reduction in the feed allowance might not act directly on the sow's organism, but indirectly through reduced exposure of the mammary complexes due to decreased amounts of faeces and urine contaminating the lying area. Information on the actual factors leading to the manifestation of mastitis in sows is widely lacking and further research is desirable.

The absorption of endotoxins from gram-negative bacteria was proposed as an explanation for early lactation problems. Indeed, some sows (< 33 %) with problem litters are positive for circulant endotoxins (Morkoc, 1983; Pejsak, 1989). The origin of these endotoxins remains unclear but may be a urinary tract inflammation, mastitis, uterine infection or the intestine. Factors that have been reported to influence the incidence of MMA or postpartum agalactia include abrupt transfer of sows to the farrowing crates (Bäckström, 1984), induction of parturition (Cerne, 1981; Holtz, 1983), timing of introduction of ad libitum feeding after farrowing (Neil, 1996) and feed allowance during late gestation (Göransson, 1989). Other procedures, such as washing the sows and the use of disinfectants in the farrowing rooms, were reported to be associated with lower pre-weaning mortality (Ravel, 1996) and a lower incidence of chronic mastitis in sows, respectively. The use of slatted floors in farrowing pens was also associated with a decreased risk of chronic mastitis in sows (Hultén, 2004). It is apparent from studies dealing with the occurrence of PDS that the causes are multifactorial and that several factors may therefore influence the prevalence of PDS in herds. Nevertheless, studies did not test the risk of occurrence of PDS in a multivariable way and were mainly focused at the sow rather than at the herd level.

Penetration of the antibiotic at the site of action

As we have seen in the introductory chapter, pharmacokinetics enables us to predict the blood or plasma concentration of a drug after its administration, but it does not allow us to know the concentrations in the other tissues of the organism at the same kinetic times, unless tissue samples are also taken. The treatment of sows affected by this syndrome is challenging as several organs may be affected at the same time. The penetration of antimicrobials will therefore be analysed in the mammary gland and in the genital and urinary tract.

PENETRATION IN THE MAMMARY GLAND

Mammary infections in species of veterinary interest can be treated by administering antimicrobials either by intramammary or intramuscular route. Unfortunately, these substances can only be administered by the intramuscular route in sows due to the anatomical conformation of the mammary gland in these animals.

In general, the ideal drug to be administered by systemic route for the treatment of mastitis should be a weak base and fat-soluble. In addition, it should have a high bioavailability after its intramuscular administration and a low binding rate to plasma proteins. The rate of transfer of the drug from the blood to the milk is directly proportional to the gradient of concentration of the drug that it is not bound to plasma proteins. Another important factor that determines the capacity of a drug to pass through the membranes is its degree of dissociation. The cellular membrane acts as a semi-permeable membrane that does not allow the flow of ionised (hydrophilic) molecules. Only the non-ionised molecules can pass through the lipid cellular membranes (depending on their liposolubility) and the passage will continue until the osmotic pressure is the same on both sides of the membrane or until the same number of non-ionised molecules are present on each side of the membrane or cellular wall. This parameter (degree of ionisation of the drug) depends on its acid dissociation constant (pKa) and on the pH of the medium. The plasma pH is constant (close to 7.4), while the pH of milk is much more variable. Indeed, the pH of normal milk ranges from 6.4 to 6.6 in cows, while the milk from a quarter with mastitis can reach values of up to 7.4 (Ziv, 1980). Similar values could be expected for sows although less information is available in the literature in comparison with the data about cows. The Henderson-Hasselbach equation relates the degree of dissociation of a molecule in the organism with the pKa acid dissociation constant of the molecule and the pH of the medium it is in (Aramayona, 1996):

For an acid: Log (non ionised/ionised) = pKa – pH

For a base: Log (ionised/non-ionised) = pKa – pH

As an example, Figure 1 shows the non-ionised and ionised fraction of penethamate hydriodide in plasma and milk of healthy cows after its intramuscular administration.

Another point that should be taken into account to assess the transfer of any drug to an organ or system is the vascularisation of the organ. The udder is highly vascularised since it requires the passage of 500 litres of blood to "produce" one litre of milk in cows. This characteristic facilitates the passage of drugs through the blood-milk barrier (Erskine, 2003). Taking into account the principles previously exposed, Table 1 gives a classification of the main antimicrobials according to their distribution in the mammary gland of cows after their administration by intramuscular route (Gruet, 2001).

Unfortunately, there is little information available in the scientific literature about the penetration of antimicrobials in sows, but it seems fair

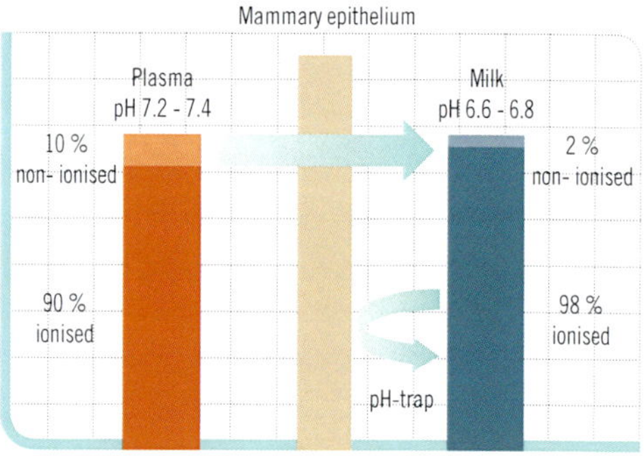

Figure 1. Graphic representation of the ionised and non-ionised fraction of penethamate hydriodide in plasma and milk of healthy cows after the administration of this drug by intramuscular route.

to think that the penetration of antimicrobials in sows is similar to the penetration observed in cows. The rabbit has also been used as a model to study the penetration of antimicrobials in milk from an experimental point of view. A study confirmed that enrofloxacin has a high degree of penetration in the milk of lactating rabbits (Aramayona, 1996) after its intramuscular administration (Fig. 2), as has been also observed in cows (Gruet, 2001).

PENETRATION IN THE URINARY TRACT

The objective of the antibiotic treatment in the case of a urinary tract infection is to inhibit bacterial growth and, if possible, destroy the bacteria present in the urine as well as in the tissues of the urinary bladder and/or the kidney in order to avoid any complications such as abscesses, septicaemia and formation of calculi. The bacteria responsible for these conditions come from the skin or the gastrointestinal tract and are able to "progress" through the urinary tract and cross the natural defence barriers involved (Dowling, 1996).

Since the 1960s, the efficacy of antibiotics for the control of urinary infections is believed to be associated with the presence of very high concentrations of these drugs in the urine of patients. However, this statement is currently under revision as, for example, the fact that high concentrations of antibiotics in urine are sufficient to guarantee efficacy in the treatment of pyelonephritis has been questioned. Many antibiotics are excreted in active form by renal route. The concentration of these drugs in urine is 100 to 1,000 times as high as their plasma concentration at the same kinetic time. The excretion of drugs through the kidney is a complex process that involves the secretion and reabsorption of these drugs in different parts of the nephron depending on their molecular structure, their pKa and the pH in the tubule (Scaglione, 2006; Fridmot-Moller, 2002b). Figure 3 shows a classification of the different antimicrobials depending on their renal excretion. Since the excretion of these antimicrobials by renal route is high, we can assume that the concentrations of these drugs in urine will also be high.

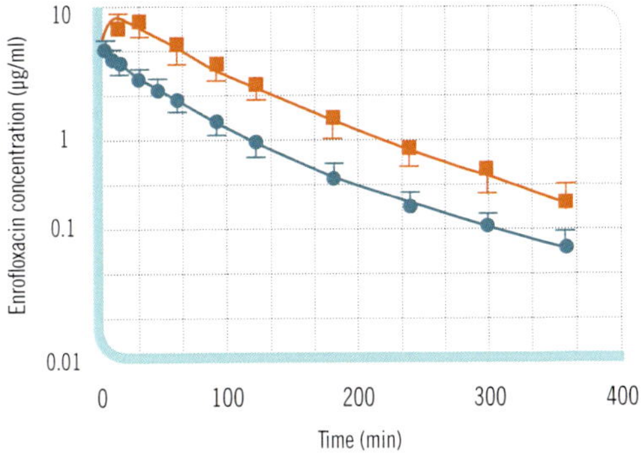

Figure 2. Semilogarithmic plot of mean ± SD concentration versus time for enrofloxacin in milk (■) and plasma (●) after IV administration of enrofloxacin (7.5 mg/kg body weight) to 6 lactating rabbits.

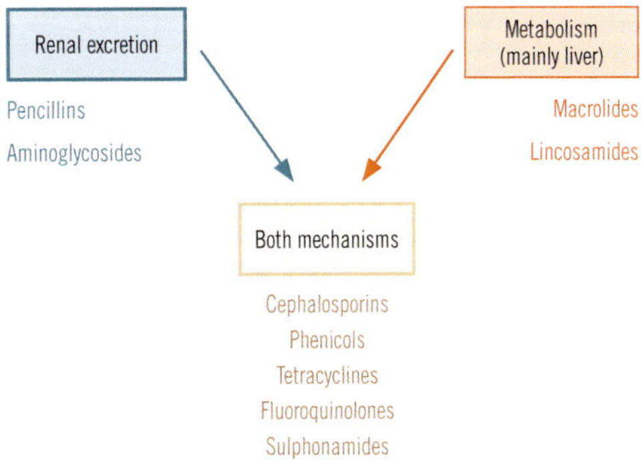

Figure 3. Characteristics of the different antimicrobials depending on their main way of elimination: metabolism versus renal excretion.

The fact that there is a very high concentration of antibiotic at the level of the tubule does not mean that this phenomenon also occurs in the kidney tissue. In fact, various authors have described that the concentration of both acid (e.g. penicillin) and basic antibiotics (e.g. trimethoprim) in the interstitial fluid of the renal medulla and cortex is similar to the plasma concentration at the same kinetic time. Other authors have come to the same conclusion since the concentration of antibiotics in kidney homogenate (including blood, renal tubule and renal tissue) is very similar to their concentration in plasma. The only antibiotics that are an exception to this general rule are aminoglycosides. These substances have a much higher concentration at tissue level than in plasma due to the fact that they bind selectively to cells of the proximal tubule epithelium (Fridmot-Moller, 2002).

As previously explained, many antibiotics concentrate in the urine. Therefore, the internal wall of the urinary bladder will be exposed to high concentrations of these substances that can significantly reduce the number of bacteria present in the lumen. However, if a bacterial infection needs to be treated at the level of an organ (tissues), the concentration of antibiotic present in the urine is irrelevant and the drug must pass from the blood to the tissues that form the urinary bladder in order to be effective.

In conclusion, it is a mistake to assume that the tissue concentration is the same as the plasma concentration at any kinetic time. On the other hand, it is very important to know the tissue concentration as it is the concentration of antimicrobial that is present in the target organ(s). When dealing with the treatment of an infection in any organ (and the urinary system is not an exception), it is essential to know where the pathogen is located exactly. Thus, the presence of high concentrations of antibiotics in urine is important to control the number of bacteria that are present at this site. However, the concentration of antibiotic present in the renal tissue can be comparable to its plasma concentration at the same kinetic times. This concentration of antibiotic in the renal tissue will be a key element to evaluate the efficacy of antibiotics in the control of bacterial nephritis.

PENETRATION IN THE GENITAL TRACT

The use of antimicrobials to treat infections of the genital tract is widely accepted, mainly in the case of metritis (Presscot, 2000). The rationale behind this therapeutic approach is to reduce the number of pathogens in the uterine cavity and consequently mitigate the associated inflammation, to enhance the local immune defense, and to facilitate endometrial repair for a faster return to a normal uterine status. Intrauterine administration of antibiotics is expected to reach a higher antibiotic concentration in the endometrium compared with systemic administration and it is the usual way to administer antimicrobials for this indication in cows and mares (Bretzlaff, 1987). A large portion of cows with clinical endometritis cure spontaneously without treatment. Cure rates defined by the absence of vaginal purulent discharge of 77 % and 63 % were reported 14 and 21 days after the first examination, respectively. These high cure rates most likely reflect the natural processes of healing during the uterine involution and may minimise the need for treatment of clinical endometritis. However, spontaneous cure of vaginal discharge does not imply increased reproductive performance and return to normal fertility. Thus, the need to treat the condition should not be underestimated (Lefevbre, 2012).

In the field of obstetrics and gynaecology, the transfer of antibiotics to the genital organs has hardly been studied as it is very difficult to examine this transfer in affected animals. There are very few reports in the world literature concerning the transfer of drugs to the lochia. However, it is important to have data about the transfer of antibiotics to the lochia for the prophylaxis and treatment of postpartum endometritis. In a study, cefpodoxime exhibited good transfer from the blood vessels to the lochia in both the uterine cavity and the vagina of women. Furthermore, cefpodoxime concentrations in the uterine cavity were similar to those observed in the vagina. Therefore, sampling of the lochia in the vagina may be a safer but equally accurate alternative to sampling of the lochia in the uterine cavity for the measurement of the drug concentrations in the lochia (Takasugi, 1996). Figure 4 shows the concentration of this cephalosporin in the genital tract and in plasma at the same time.

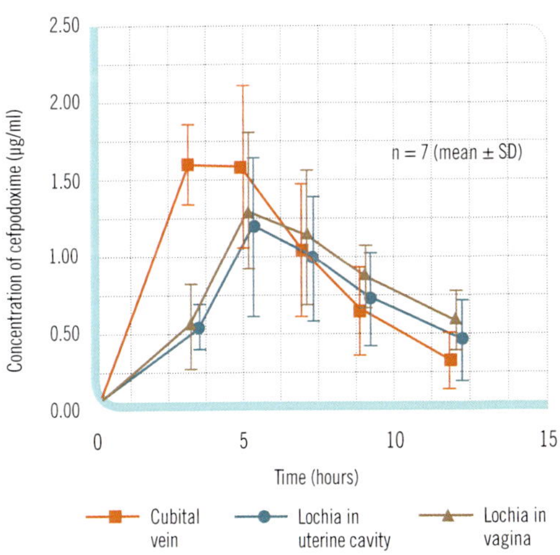

Figure 4. Changes in cefpodoxime concentrations after the oral administration of 200 mg of cefpodoxime. The cefpodoxime concentrations in the lochia gradually increased and became greater than those in the serum of cubital venous blood 9 h after cefpodoxime administration. Vertical bars represent standard deviations.

Trovafloxacin and meropenem also achieve reasonable concentrations in the endometrium although the ratio endometrial concentration/ plasma concentration was only 0.6 for the first drug and 0.4 for the second (Martens, 1998; Gall, 1997). Unfortunately, there is little data available about the penetration of antibiotics in the genital tract of sows. It seems fair to assume that similar ratios could be achieved in sows for cephalosporins and quinolones taking into account data from other species.

Treatment of MMA syndrome in sows

Description of the clinical case in swine

CLINICAL HISTORY

- Sow production unit of 2000 animals.
- An all-in-all-out system is applied in each farrowing room.
- Herd performance before the clinical outbreak: optimum.
- Age of the animals: adult sows.

CLINICAL SIGNS OBSERVED

- Some sows show signs of anorexia and depression (Fig. 5).
- The mammary glands of some sows are warm to the touch and swollen, with a blotched appearance (Figs. 6 and 7).
- When many glands are involved, the sows often go off feed and have high rectal temperatures (> 40 °C).
- A high piglet mortality rate can be observed in the litter of the affected sows, probably due to starvation and hypothermia.
- The urine of the sows looks normal and no discharge has been observed through the vulva.

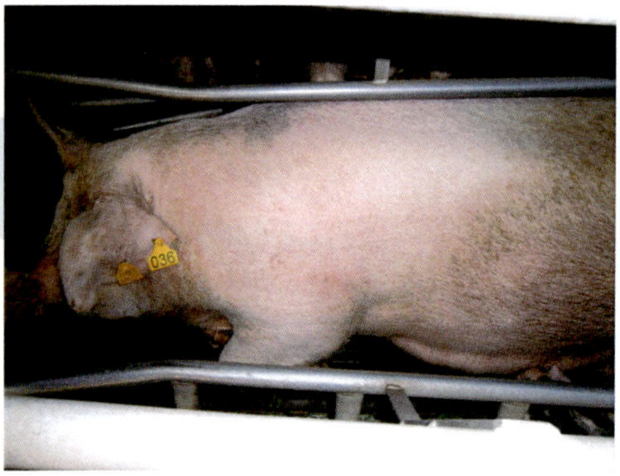

Figure 5

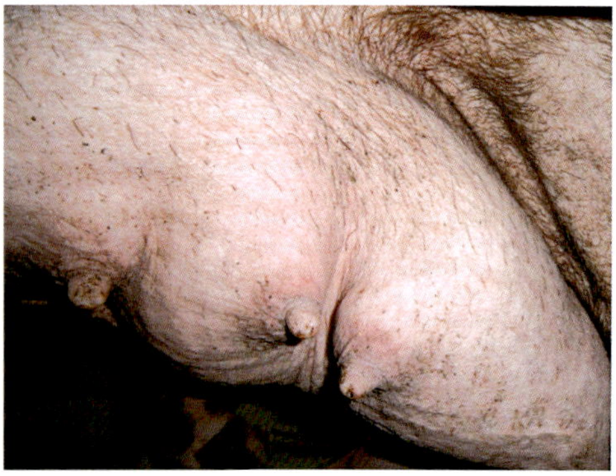

Figure 6

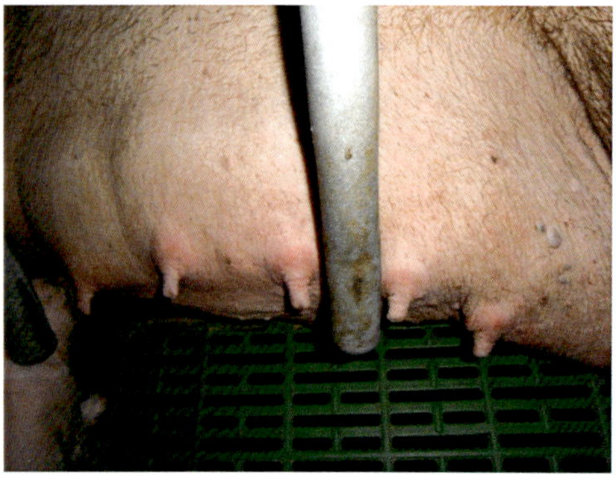

Figure 7

PRESUMPTIVE DIAGNOSIS

- Sows affected of post-partum dysgalactia syndrome where mastitis seems to be the main clinical problem.

INITIAL TREATMENT

Symptomatic

- A non-steroidal anti-inflammatory drug (NSAID) was administered by intramuscular route in a single dose.

Aetiologic

- An antibiotic should be administered to control this bacterial infection. This point will be analysed further on.

Critical review of the treatment

SYMPTOMATIC

ANTI-ENDOTOXIC DRUGS

Many clinical signs observed in sows (depression, fever and even tachypnoea and tachycardia) have their origin in the endotoxic disease (presence of circulating toxins) associated with this condition. It has been demonstrated that the use of NSAIDs seems to have a beneficial effect on the health of affected sows as an adjuvant therapy in the treatment of MMA (Klopfenstein, 2006).

AETIOLOGIC. CRITICAL REVIEW OF THE APPLICATION OF ANTIBIOTICS IN THE TREATMENT

NEED TO USE ANTIMICROBIALS

There is a generalised consensus in the consulted literature about the need to use antibiotics to treat clinical cases of MMA (Prescott, 2000). The antibiotics most commonly used in this case belong to the families of quinolones (enrofloxacin, marbofloxacin and danofloxacin) and β-lactams (amoxicillin and cephalosporins) taking into account the bacterial species to be treated.

Therapeutic approach

The elements that should be taken into account are the following:

1. The infection is located in the mammary gland, urinary tract and, less frequently, in the genital tract.
2. The selected dosage regimen must reach sufficient concentrations at the sites of action so they can inhibit bacterial growth and be maintained for a sufficient period of time.
3. The antimicrobial must exert a very fast action since the disease evolves very quickly.

An antibiotic should be chosen taking into account these considerations. In this case, the antimicrobial must be active against *Escherichia coli* and microorganisms of the *Staphylococcus* genera, since they are the most frequent bacteria involved in this syndrome (Kemper, 2009). As seen in the first chapter, the antimicrobial susceptibility of bacteria is usually measured with the MIC value. The MIC values of a list of antimicrobials belonging to a wide range of families that can be used against *Escherichia coli* are included in Table 2.

Table 3 shows the MIC values of a list of antimicrobials belonging to a wide range of families that can be used against *Staphylococcus hyicus*. This microorganism is the most common pathogen isolated from sows with mastitis within the genus *Staphylococcus* (Kemper, 2009).

The MIC of amoxicillin against *Staphylococcus hyicus* is 8 µg/ml. However, the MIC value of amoxicillin against this bacterium is 0.5 µg/ml when amoxicillin and clavulanic acid are jointly administered.

The second element that needs to be known is the concentration of the antimicrobial that will be reached at the site of action. In this case, the site of action is the mammary gland, urinary and possibly the genital tract. The degree of penetration of the antimicrobials that may be used to treat clinical cases of MMA in sows after parenteral administration can be seen in Table 4.

PK/PD parameter for a concentration-dependent antibiotic

A concentration-dependent antibiotic is an antibiotic with an effect on microorganisms that depends on their concentration. In the case of marbofloxacin, the Cmax/MIC and AUC/MIC ratios are the PK/PD parameters that best correlate with clinical efficacy. An AUC/MIC ratio value of 100 is taken as a reference in this case, since there is no precise information available in the literature about the PK/PD parameter values in the treatment of specific diseases in veterinary medicine (Guyonnet, 2003; Apley, 2005).

Figure 8 shows the marbofloxacin concentration in plasma after the intramuscular administration of a dose of 2 mg/kg body weight of this antibiotic in sows. The Cmax and AUC value are close to 1 µg/ml and 15.32 µg/ml/hr, respectively. Thus, if the AUC is calculated from the concentration of antibiotic in

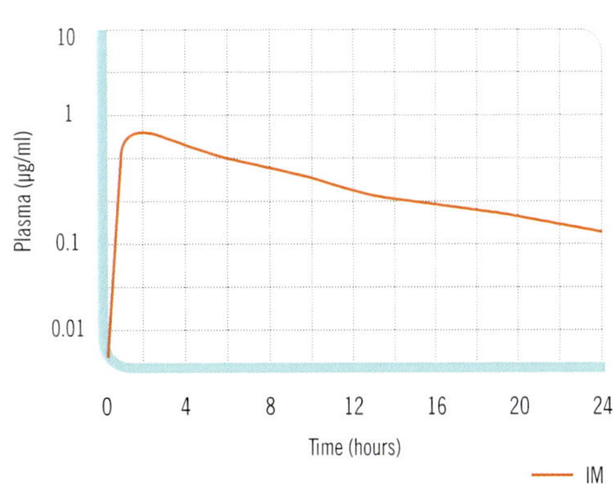

Figure 8. Plasma kinetics following the IM administration of a single dose of 2 mg/kg marbofloxacin in pigs.

plasma (AUC_{plasma}), the AUC/MIC ratio value in this case is 73 (15.32/0.21) for marbofloxacin and *Escherichia* coli. This value is under the threshold value (AUC/MIC = 100) usually accepted for quinolones. However, quinolones have a good degree of penetration in milk (Fig. 2). In studies carried out in rabbits, the AUC_{milk}/AUC_{plasma} ratio had a value of 2-3 and 4-5 for enrofloxacin and ciprofloxacin, respectively (Aramayona, 1996). Curiously, the AUC_{milk}/AUC_{plasma} ratio for marbofloxacin in the case of cows (Schneider, 2004) was close to 1 (Fig. 9), suggesting that marbofloxacin seems to have a low transfer rate from plasma to milk in comparison with other quinolones. Unfortunately, there is no data available about the penetration of marbofloxacin in sows and the exact PK/PD parameters cannot be calculated. Nevertheless, if we consider that marbofloxacin has a similar degree of penetration in sow's milk than in cow's milk, the AUC/MIC value will be 73.

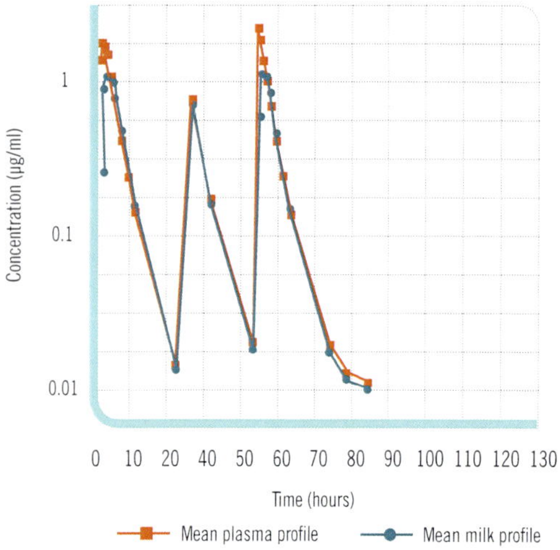

Figure 9. Mean plasma and milk concentration-time profile of marbofloxacin in the dairy cow after repeated intramuscular administrations at a dose rate of 2 mg/kg every 24 h for 3 days.

However, if it is assumed that marbofloxacin has a similar penetration in sow's milk as in the milk of rabbits (a very conservative estimation), the AUC_{milk}/MIC value will be 146 (2* 15.32/0.21).

In conclusion, the AUC/MIC ratio for marbofloxacin could reach a value between 73 and 146 when treating an *Escherichia coli* infection in the mammary glands of sows. Given the results obtained and considering an AUC/MIC ratio value of 100 as an indicator of efficacy, the treatment can be expected to be effective. These results have been corroborated by clinical trials in which the efficacy of the treatment with marbofloxacin for this disease has been unequivocally confirmed.

The probability of clinical success for the antimicrobials that may be used for the treatment of MMA can be calculated taking into account the pharmacokinetic and pharmacodynamic information available in the public domain and their pharmacokinetic properties. These can be provided by the pharmaceutical company or found in the literature.

The information provided in Table 2 and 3 is for guidance only, as each strain has its own MIC value for each antimicrobial. The PK/PD parameters of the antimicrobials that may be used should therefore be calculated for each clinical case and the result should be taken into account to optimise the therapy and choose the best antimicrobial option (see Fig. 14 in chapter 2). In addition, in order to choose an appropriate antimicrobial agent, swine practitioners should know the efficacy of the molecule (previously analysed), the current regulations on the use of antimicrobials in their country and the history of the herd.

Table 1. Distribution of antimicrobials in the mammary gland after their administration by intramuscular route in cows (Gruet, 2001).

Distribution	Drugs
Good	Quinolones Sulphanilamide Erythromycin Tylosin Spiramycin Lincomycin Trimethoprim Tiamulin
Limited	Penicillin G Ampicillin Amoxicillin Tetracycline Cephalosporins
Poor	Spectinomycin Dihydrostreptomycin Neomycin Kanamycin Gentamicin Polymyxin

Table 2. MIC of antimicrobials for the treatment of an *Escherichia coli* infection (Burch, 2007, and author's own data).

Antimicrobial	MIC range (µg/ml)	MIC_{90} (µg/ml)	Epidemiological cut-off (µg/ml)	Clinical cut-off (µg/ml)
Danofloxacin	0.03-1	0.125	-	-
Enrofloxacin	0.03-1	0.25	0.06	2
Marbofloxacin	-	0.210		
Ampicillin	1-64	64	8	16
Amoxicillin + Clavulanic acid	2-64	8	16	16
Sulfamethoxazole + Trimethoprim	0.5-8	8	1	4
Sulfadiazine + Trimethoprim	0.31- > 40	1.25*	-	-
Neomycin	2-64	64	4	8
Spectinomycin	8-256	256	32	64
Colistin sulphate	2-4	2	4	8

* MIC_{50}

Table 3. MIC of antimicrobials for the treatment of a *Staphylococcus hyicus* infection (Wegener, 1994; Futagawa-Saito, 2009).

	Wegener et al., 1994		Futagawa-Saito, 2009	
Antimicrobial	MIC range (µg/ml)	MIC_{90} (µg/ml)	MIC range (µg/ml)	MIC_{90} (µg/ml)
Enrofloxacin	0.13-0.5	0.25	-	-
Ofloxacin	-	-	0.25-1	-
Ampicillin	< 0.03-2	0.5	0.12- >16	-
Penicillin	-	-	< 0.06- > 8	
Cephalosporins (cefuroxime)	-	-	< 0.5-2	
Streptomycin	1- > 64	> 64	-	-
Phenicols (chloramphenicol)	-	-	4-64	-

Table 4. Penetration of antimicrobials in the site of action.

Antimicrobial group	Mammary gland	Urinary tract	Genital tract
Fluoroquinolones	++/+++	+++	+/++$
Beta-lactams (no cephalosporins)	+/++*	+++	+/++*
Cephalosporins	+/++*	++/+++	++/+++*$

-, no, + low, ++ intermediate and +++ high penetration.

* Higher in inflamed tissues. $ Data from a cephalosporin and quinolone for human use.

Table 5. Probability of clinical success for antimicrobials in the treatment of MMA infections.

Antimicrobial group	PK/PD parameter and threshold value	Probability of success in the mammary gland	Probability of success in the urinary tract	Probability of success in the genital tract
Fluoroquinolones	AUC/MIC > 100 and T > MIC?$	++/+++	+++	++/+++
Cephalosporins	T > MIC	++/+++	++/+++	+/++
Beta-lactams (no cephalosporins)	T > MIC	+/++	+++	+/++
Aminoglycosides	Cmax/MIC > 10	-	+/++&	-

Probability of success: - failure, + low, ++ intermediate and +++ high.

$ A time-dependent activity has been described for gram-positive germs in the case of marbofloxacin (e.g.: *Staphylococci*).

& Be careful with renal toxicity.

Responsible use of antimicrobials in pig production

6

Responsible use of antimicrobials in pig production

6

Written in collaboration with Dr John Mackinnon

Use of antimicrobials in pig production

Why use antimicrobials in pig production?

There are three main reasons for using antimicrobials in pig production: animal health and welfare, carcass and meat quality and economics of production.

- **Animal health and welfare:**
  " Any animal which appears to be ill or injured must be cared for appropriately without delay. " (Council Directive 98/58/EC)
  European law requires that sick animals are given appropriate care. Where bacterial infections or other infectious agents with bacterial involvement are the cause of illness, appropriate care is likely to involve the use of antimicrobials. Several basic features of pig production render pig populations susceptible to epizootic and enzootic disease. These are population size in relation to space, a high potential for contact with excreta and discharges and, within groups, uniformity of age and immune status. Furthermore, there is no transplacental immunity in the pig and early gut closure to colostral immunoglobulins means that the young pig is almost entirely dependent on an adequate supply of colostrum in the first 24-36 hours of life for immune protection over the first weeks. The stress of weaning and mixing litters together increases circulating cortisol levels and, in turn, there is a potential suppressing effect on immune competence.
- **Carcass and meat quality:**
  Large quantities of meat are lost due to trimming or total carcass rejection because of the presence of abscesses, sepsis, polyserositis, etc. These conditions render meat unsuitable for human consumption and their prevalence can be reduced by an appropriate use of antimicrobials. Among the 40 potential porcine zoonoses listed by Alexander in 1998, 10 bacterial zoonoses are of significant concern. An appropriate use of antimicrobials together with proper animal management methods might help reduce carriage of these infections.
- **Economics:**
  Farming is not a charity and cost-effective food production is necessary to ensure supply at an appropriate price. In many situations, the presence of an infectious disease can determine whether a producer makes a profit or a loss. Economic loss in agriculture is one of the main causes of lack of investment, which, in turn, leads to poor conditions, poor welfare and ever increasing burdens of infection. The appropriate use of antimicrobials in situations in which a bacterial disease is endemic can help maintain efficient production (Fig. 1), but it is a myth that farmers can afford to use very large quantities of antimicrobials on a routine basis.

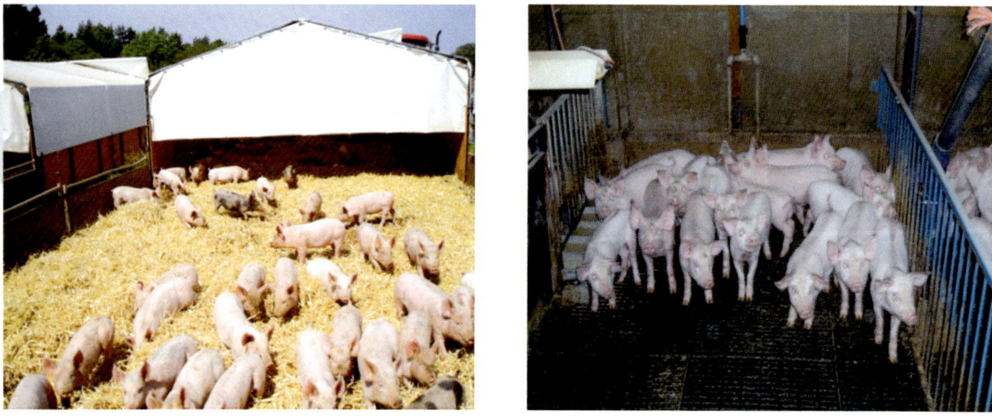

Figure 1. These animals show a good health status and efficient pig production.

How to control the use of antimicrobials in pig production?

There is some misconception amongst consumer groups that antimicrobials are widely and indiscriminately used. In a minority of cases, overuse of antibiotics may occur but it must be recognised that there are a number of legislative controls in place that aim at restricting the misuse of antimicrobials:

- **Human safety:** In Europe, the use of medicines for the treatment of food animals is governed by ***Directive 2001/82/EC***, the main aim of which is to safeguard human and animal safety. Under European (EU) legislation, antimicrobials must first be authorised for sale in the EU and secondly, they must be used within their marketing authorisation. More specifically, they must be licensed for use in pigs.
- **Veterinary prescription:** Many medicines including antimicrobials belong to the controlled category requiring a veterinary prescription or veterinary control. These establish specific limitations for safety reasons, due to the need to have specific veterinary knowledge when there is a narrow margin of safety or when there is a government policy requiring the control of a professional. In addition, various efforts are being made to subcategorise antibiotics in relation to their importance in human medicine.
- **Distribution:** There is an approved sales and distribution channel through authorised wholesalers, retailers and pharmacies. At farm level, the prescribing veterinary surgeon must be specifically appointed by the owner of the animals as the veterinary surgeon responsible for their care and treatment. Records of all treatments are required to be kept for periods of up to 5 years.
- **Monitoring:** In addition, the European Commission is actively working on an overarching European strategy on antimicrobial resistance, covering both human and animal health aspects. One important part of this strategy is to monitor the sales of veterinary antibiotics through the Surveillance of Veterinary Antimicrobial Consumption that is actually being implemented throughout Europe.

Various organisations such as the FAO, WHO and OIE hold meetings of experts to review matters pertaining to animal and human health. In 2007, a meeting was held on antimicrobials, during which antibiotics used in human health were classified as being critically important, highly important or simply important. This classification was updated in 2012. Table 1 classifies all the antimicrobial families potentially suitable to be used in veterinary medicine according to their relevance for human health. On the other hand, Table 2 summarises the formulations licensed for use in pigs in the European Union. There are variations from country to country, but it shows what is usually available. It must be highlighted that in many cases the same antimicrobials that are particularly relevant in human medicine are also similarly relevant in veterinary medicine.

Understanding antimicrobials and bacterial resistance to them

The discovery of antimicrobials began a new period in the medicine preventive programmes applied in livestock. However, it was realised that the emergence of resistant microbes could decrease the efficacy of these tools to control infectious diseases in these animals. Antimicrobial resistance was linked to the use of these drugs and it was intrinsically recognised as a modern phenomenon. However, resistance is not new; it is an ancient, naturally occurring phenomenon widespread in the environment. Many of the antibiotics we use in human and veterinary medicine are naturally produced by bacteria. Therefore, it is normal for bacteria to have resistance mechanisms in place to be protected against these substances; it is part of their inherent survival strategy. In a cave in New Mexico that had remained undisturbed for over 4 million years, bacteria were found with known and even as-yet-unknown resistance mechanisms against the most modern antibiotics, for instance daptomycin, a compound only used in human medicine (Bhullar et al., 2012). Similar findings are reported for bacteria isolated from permafrost, another environment unexposed to antibiotics currently used in human or animal medicine (D'costa, 2011). These findings clearly suggest that antibiotic resistance is a natural phenomenon that existed before the selective pressure of clinical antimicrobial use.

How does antimicrobial resistance emerge?

Bacteria become resistant by:

- Inactivating the antimicrobial.
- Modifying the target site of action of the antimicrobial.
- Reducing the accumulation of the antimicrobial within the bacterial cell.
- Replacing a component of the metabolism pathway affected by the antimicrobial.

Some bacteria are inherently tolerant of, or resistant to, some classes of antimicrobials. This type of resistance is likely to have evolved millions of years ago. However, currently, the most important resistance development mechanisms are through the acquisition of genetic material from other bacteria of the same or different species (e.g. β-lactam resistance in gram-negative bacteria). In other situations, for example with fluoroquinolones, resistance may additionally occur due to genetic mutation. A summary of the main mechanisms of resistance previously described is shown in Figure 2 and they have also been classified according to its antimicrobial family in Table 3.

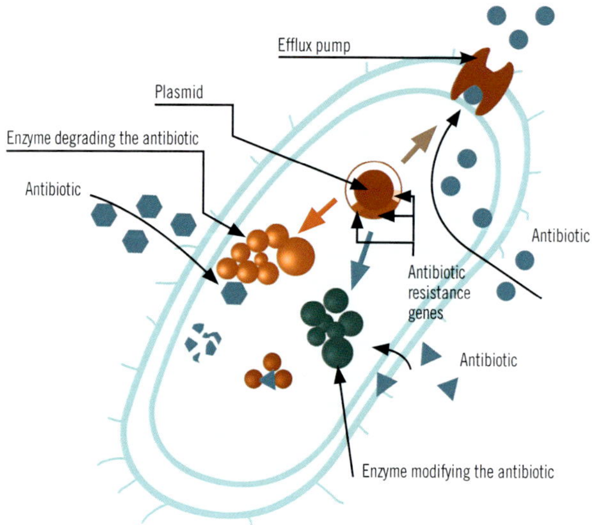

Figure 2. Common mechanisms of emergence of resistances. Image courtesy of A. Pridmore.

The genetic material responsible for antimicrobial resistance may come from a mutation in the genetic determination for sensitivity or in the acquisition of extrachromosomal DNA carrying resistance genes. These mechanisms are explained in detail below:

- **Acquisition of extrachromosomal DNA carrying a resistance gene:** Extrachromosomal DNA can be located on mobile genetic elements such as plasmids and transposons, which can be transmitted widely among bacteria; and their spread may be quite fast. This genetic material potentially carries resistance genes and codes for virulence.
- **Mutation in the genetic determinant for sensitivity:** A random mutation can occur in the genes that determine sensitivity to an antimicrobial. This is a relatively uncommon event and usually arises within the range of antimicrobial concentrations corresponding to the specific mutant selection window. This type of resistance can only be transmitted vertically to progeny by replication. It is slow to emerge and spread within the bacterial population and it tends to disappear once the antimicrobial in question has been removed.

Why is antimicrobial resistance a concern?

While the emergence of antimicrobial resistance is not surprising, it has raised concerns. The main issue in the medical field is the emergence of multi-resistance in healthcare environments as a result of prolonged exposure to antimicrobials.

- The earliest concern regarding antimicrobial resistance in human medicine was the emergence of methicillin-resistant *Staphylococcus aureus* (MRSA) because methicillin-resistant strains typically show extensive multiple resistance to a number of antimicrobials and may cause severe infections. The classification of MRSA in humans is complex because it is based on their epidemiological pattern (which may not be very closely correlated to particular strains). Human MRSA include hospital acquired (HA), community acquired (CA) MRSA and a "healthcare" associated infection: typically these are transmitted between humans by touch and poor hygiene. Livestock associated (LA) MRSA, which has the highest incidence in swine herds, is spread by contact regardless of whether antimicrobials are used or not, affecting primarily farmers, vets and meat-workers. LA-MRSA readily colonises animals but infections in both animals and humans are rare. More recently, an atypical MRSA, the so called mecC, has been identified but is still rare in both humans and animals.

- Over the last decade, the main concern in humans relates to the production of *extended-spectrum β-lactamases* (ESBLs) that confer resistance to penicillins, cephalosporins and monobactams in *Escherichia coli, Salmonella* spp. and *Klebsiella* spp. It is important to note that the main cause of human infections with ESBL-producing bacteria is a result of antimicrobial use in humans. In livestock, ESBL bacteria are often commensal and there is concern that foodborne spread might lead to zoonotic infection or gene transfer to human pathogens. More recently, the concern has been focused on carbapenemases in human hospital infections: these have been isolated only rarely and sporadically from animal samples (carbapenem-type antibiotics are not licensed in animals and are extremely unlikely to be used in livestock due to their high cost).
- Major concerns also exist regarding multi-resistant tuberculosis and gonorrhoea in humans.

The concern about antimicrobial resistance comes largely from the human side of the debate and, obviously, the question of risk to human health must be the centre of the analysis. While there continues to be debate, **most of the risk of antimicrobial resistance for human health comes from the use of these antimicrobials in human beings.** Nevertheless, it must be also accepted that a small part of this risk may result from the use of antimicrobials in animals. Figure 3 represents the global epidemiology of antimicrobial resistance taking into account a wide range of factors and their relationships. It seems that the global transmission of resistant bacteria has increased with the advent of widespread international travel and cross-border trade in food and animals. **In any case, the risk of acquisition of antimicrobial resistance in humans due to the use of these substances in animals is estimated to be very low.** For example, according to Hurd (2010), for macrolide antibiotics there is a one in ten million chance for a human patient to suffer from diarrhoea for a longer period of time (one or two days) as a result of a resistance originated in the animal population and causing treatment failure in humans. To put this into perspective, the chances of being killed in an air crash are about the same.

Antimicrobial use and resistance

For many years, ecological studies have shown a link between the frequency of resistance and the use of antimicrobials. This has been observed both in hospital and in community environments. Moreover, the same correlation has been seen in agriculture, in particular in the cattle industry (Levy, 1997; Shryock, 2010). The observed increase in the incidence of resistance is an expected result. By contrast, when antimicrobial use is reduced or abolished, a decrease of resistance prevalence may occur, but is less obvious or not achieved (Sundqvist, 2010; Andersson, 2011).

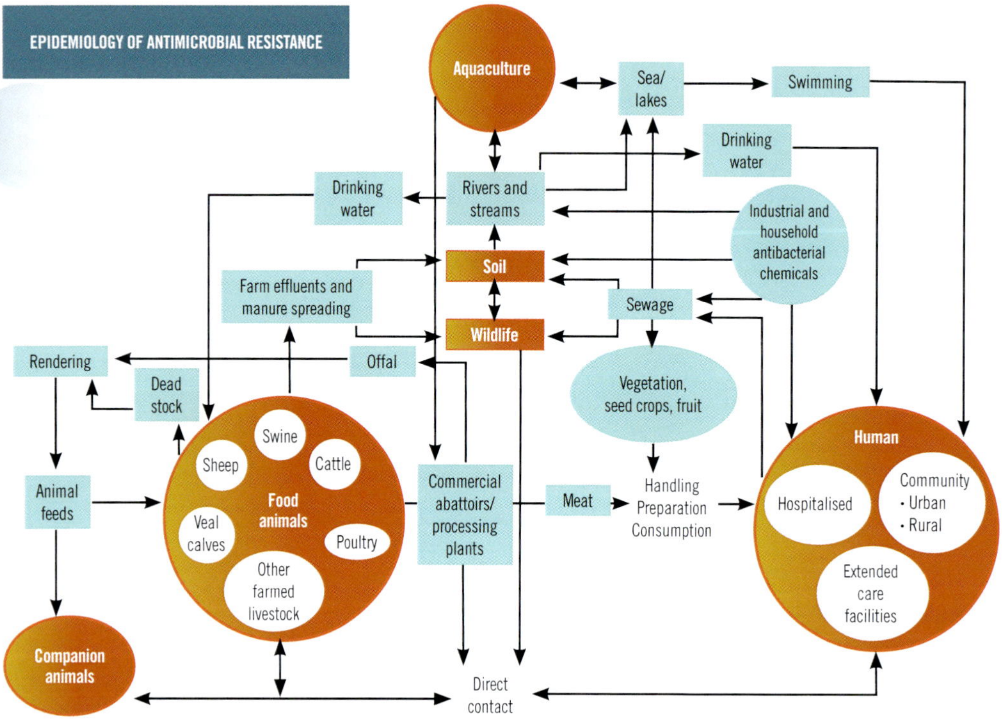

Figure 3. The pathways of resistance transmission (Prescott, 2000).

Since the introduction of antimicrobials into medical practice, the increase in the frequency of resistance has become a common collateral effect of their use. First anecdotal reports were followed by a huge body of evidence for a vicious circle in which the introduction of a new antimicrobial agent is followed by the emergence of resistance. The subsequently needed development of new compounds that are not affected by previous resistance mechanisms will lead, sooner or later, to the selection of new resistances. A supranational multicentre study has demonstrated that European countries with a higher consumption of antimicrobials in hospitals have a higher incidence of methicillin-resistant *S. aureus* (MRSA) (Mackenzie, 2007). In some instances, a time-series analysis is required to observe a relationship between consumption and resistance.

Global reduction of antimicrobial use does not always result in a decline of resistance although it has been observed many times under field conditions. For instance, a nonreverting trimethoprim/sulphonamide resistance has been observed in *E. coli* despite a clear decrease in the use of these antibiotics in a community setting (Sundqvist, 2010). This lack of reversion to susceptibility can be due to the absence of a significant fitness cost of the resistance traits or to their permanent fixation (e.g. on an integron) in the bacterial population (Cantón, 2003[a]; Cantón, 2011). Antibiotic stewardship programmes have been in part designed to try and curtail resistances once they have arisen (Tamma, 2011). Interestingly, these studies have also confirmed important difficulties in curtailing resistance once this event has occurred (Rahal, 2002). In many cases, this is due to the coresistance phenomenon: another antimicrobial class is also unable to kill or suppress bacterial growth because the targeted microorganism is insensitive to the new compound as well.

Hazards, risks and hazard management

Antimicrobial resistance constitutes a potential hazard to human or animal health, and risk is the probability of this hazard to occur (i.e. a human being or animal suffers damages due to treatment failure of a resistant bacteria). The principles of hazard analysis and critical control points (HACCP) can be applied to the hazard of the resistant organisms present on a farm. There are many steps in the food chain involving different procedures where controls aimed at reducing the risk of transfer of antimicrobial resistance might be applied. These points have been marked with different colours in Figures 4 and 5.

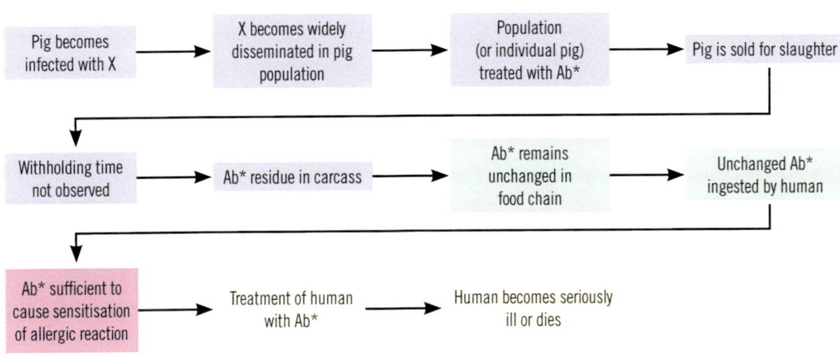

Figure 4

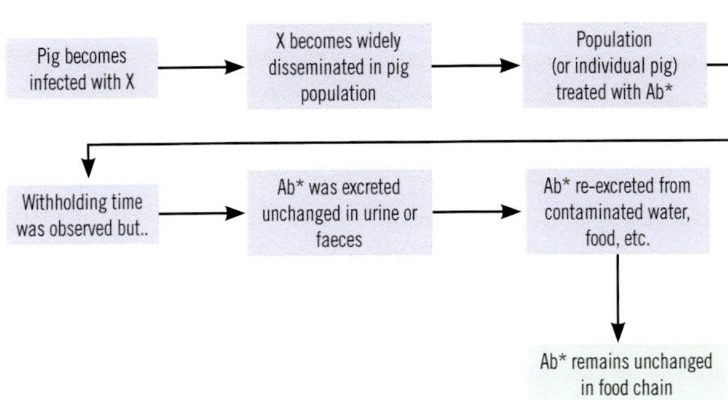

Figure 5

The various steps have been colour-coded according to the HACCP principles.
Purple: Factors under control of veterinary surgeons and farmers.
Green: Factors under control of food processors and people preparing food.
Pink: Chance effects that may be influenced by lifestyle, environment, etc.
Yellow: Factors under the control of physicians and their patients.

What are these principles in relation with antimicrobial resistance?

1. Carry out hazard analysis: identify hazards and assess the associated risk.
2. Identify Critical Control points (CCPs), points at which hazards can be controlled.
3. Establish critical limits: What is unacceptable? Establish a monitoring system: Is the critical point under control?
4. Establish procedures for corrective action: Define actions if the critical point is not under control.
5. Establish procedures to verify hazard control, like random checks and sampling.
6. Keep documentation of procedures and records of actions and outcomes open to external audit.

Finally, the different points where a control can be applied to decrease the spread of antimicrobial resistance not only in animals but also in humans are summarised in Table 4. The person responsible for each control point is also specified.

Responsible use of antimicrobials

Reducing the need for antibiotics

The starting point in the responsible use of antimicrobials is to reduce the need for them:

- **Prevent disease entry:** The first principle is to prevent disease entry into the herd. This requires sourcing healthy animals, good biosecurity procedures that include proper isolation and monitoring, and a comprehensive and appropriate vaccination programme designed by the herd veterinary surgeon.
- **Prevent clinical emergence of dormant infection:** It is surprising how an infection can remain dormant for long periods of time without any clinical signs and without the need for antimicrobials, a typical example being swine dysentery. Many herds can live with an endemic disease providing high standards of nutrition, management and environmental control.
- **Control endemic disease:** Endemic disease must also be controlled by managing pig-flow, with all-in-all-out principles combined with adherence to effective cleaning and disinfection protocols. This may require modifications of the site to manage pig flow, but the process is likely to be cost-effective in controlling the infection. At the same time, vectors of disease such as rats, mice and flies must be eliminated or comprehensively controlled.
- **Control dissemination of disease on farm:** It is easy to spread a disease by handling pigs for procedures such as vaccination, ear-tagging, injections, tail-docking, teeth-clipping and fostering, etc. All of these management tasks must be done hygienically and according to sensible protocols aimed at reducing the spread of the infection.
- **Break infection cycles** to prevent the spread of resistant bacteria: Beside the all-in-all-out principle, buildings should also be disinfected at the earliest opportunity. Different types of disinfectants should be used in rotation and any equipment potentially contaminated with pathogens such as drinkers, feed troughs, etc., should be cleaned and disinfected to prevent the potential maintenance and carryover of resistant bacteria in the environment.

Making the right choice: treatment and route of administration

Making the right choice of antimicrobials and route of administration is essential for their responsible use. Treatments should be justified professionally and instructions must be explicit, possibly as part of the herd health plan:

- **Follow legislation and use products according to their label:** European legislation governs the choice of treatment to a great degree and in the first instance this should be an antimicrobial that has been licensed for the given indication in the species to be treated.
- **Use previous clinical and diagnostic experience:** Decisions are influenced by the veterinary surgeon's previous clinical experience and understanding of the nature of the infection to be treated. It is always helpful to isolate and identify the pathogen and to obtain a sensitivity profile but in practice, time is not on the side of the vet and decisions have to be made before laboratory results are available, hence the importance of previous clinical experience and knowing the sensitivity patterns of pathogens within a herd.
- **Determine a dosage regimen in case of cascade use:** Using pharmacokinetic and pharmacodynamic data, the aim should be to determine the dosage regimen that brings about bactericidal activity. In practice, one is largely dependent on the guidance given in the product data sheet or in the summary of product characteristics (SPC) but the first principles should be used if appropriate data is available.
- **Cost factors:** A high cost can be an obstacle to compliance. It is important to ensure that full courses of treatment are completed and, therefore, product cost might influence choice.
- **Consider elimination of antibiotic:** Consideration should of course be given to appropriate withholding times to safeguard consumer safety.
- **Route of administration:** Injection is by far the best option since it provides an accurate dose to the individual pig. In diseased animals, a treatment based on water medication will probably ensure a better compliance than via feed.

Monitoring the use of antimicrobials

The use of antimicrobials should be monitored on the farm using various tools such as:

- **Record keeping:** There are statutory requirements for records of treatments to be kept for up to five years, to include animal identity, dates of treatment, doses used, etc. Some national schemes require regular reconciliation of the amounts of antimicrobials used with the quantities prescribed or purchased.
- **Calculating amounts:** Calculating the amounts of antimicrobials used can be done in a variety of ways such as the number of treatment days per animal, the average quantities used per pig slaughtered or the number of pigs treated by class or weight range over time. Any form of calculation should be standardised on the amounts of active ingredient, not on the amounts of commercial product. This point is critical when the use in different European countries is compared following the European community legislation.

Early detection and individual treatment of pigs

The concept of treating pigs as individuals within herds rather than using a blanket approach and taking the herd as a whole is not new. This approach is an application of common sense combined with good veterinary practice and a responsible attitude towards the use of antimicrobials. Furthermore, it can help pig farmers find solutions to their most common issues:

- **Becoming more effective:** Desrosiers and Martineau (1984) already showed 29 years ago that pleuropneumonia in finishing pigs can be more effectively controlled by individually targeted parenteral treatment accompanied by appropriate environmental management than it can by metaphylactic feed or water medication.
- **Protecting young pigs:** In young pigs particularly, immunity is not fully developed and some features of pig production increase the risk of disease: relatively large populations in relation to space, contact with excreta and discharges, and uniformity of age and immune status render populations uniformly susceptible to certain infections.
- **Making monitoring more accurate:** Treating pigs individually can make the monitoring of the use of antimicrobials and the recording of the clinical outcome easier and more accurate, by allowing calculations of treatment days or average doses given per animal over time. Eventually, the cost benefits could be calculated from the production results in terms of growth rate and feed conversion.
- **Following EU requirements:** The individual treatment of pigs fulfils the legal requirements for the treatment of sick animals as laid down by Council Directives 98/58/EC and 2008/120/EC. Animals must be inspected at least once a day or as appropriate and any individual found sick must be treated without delay. Treatment and mortality records must also be kept.
- **Animal welfare:** Treating pigs individually can help improve animal welfare on a day-to-day basis by documenting the prevalence and incidence of diseases and the clinical outcome of the treatments. The so-called "tip of the iceberg" conditions are lameness, behavioural issues such as tail-biting and injuries.
- Individual Pig Care is a swine herd management programme that focuses on the profitable rearing of pigs, respecting welfare, optimising the correct use of medicines and utilising skilled stockmen. By providing, without extra work, information on clinical, therapeutical and husbandry profiles, Individual Pig Care is an innovative and differentiating system for swine vets and producers to help them being more efficient, using anti-infectives in a more responsible way.

Impact of infection and its control

- **Control of economical impact:** For pig producers, it is important to demonstrate the economics of infection control through the individual treatment of pigs. This can be done by evaluating the production parameters, calculating the value of reduced mortality, days to slaughter and pen occupancy; and finally by calculating the return on investment.
- **Food safety and carcass:** Microbial infections that may be controlled by an effective use of antimicrobials can cause carcasses to be trimmed or rejected at the slaughterhouse, with dire economic consequences for producers. The main lesions observed in the carcasses are abscesses, peritonitis, pleurisy, pneumonia, pyaemia, septic arthritis, oedema and emaciation.
- **Meat hygiene control:** The potential for carriage of zoonotic agents is an important consideration in meat hygiene controls.

Zoonotic agents such as *Erysipelothrix*, *Salmonella* spp., *Campylobacter* spp., or *Yersinia enterocolitica*, could possibly be limited with an effective use of antimicrobials together with hygiene control and good husbandry.

- **Consumer protection:** In terms of consumer protection, a formal and responsible approach to the use of antimicrobials should reduce the risk of emergence of bacterial resistance through its targeted approach to treatment. Furthermore, respecting the withdrawal period avoids unsafe antimicrobial residues.

Practical recommendation for a prudent use of antimicrobials

Several institutions have published recommendations for a prudent use of antimicrobials under field conditions (Federation of Veterinarians of Europe and American Veterinary Medical Association). They have been included in the text literally (cursive text) and can be summarised as follow:

1. **Never prescribe antimicrobials without doing an examination and diagnosis:**
   "You should only prescribe the correct dosage of antimicrobials following an examination and clinical diagnosis. You should also do sensitivity testing whenever possible. Always evaluate how well the treatment has worked afterwards."
2. **Work with your clients to minimise and eliminate the need for antimicrobials:**
   "Plans should outline how farmers will ensure their animals' health and provide effective biosecurity. Prevention is essential for all animals."
3. **Use diagnostic tests, including susceptibility tests, as much as possible:**
   "Do a diagnostic test before prescribing antimicrobials, if possible on the farm. Even if you need to begin treatment immediately, it is still useful to do a test to confirm your diagnosis, or to be able to change your treatment as a result of laboratory findings."
4. **Use antimicrobials correctly:**
   "Limit the use of antimicrobials as much as possible: only use them for sick animals or animals at risk; minimise routine use (for example, do not regularly use antimicrobials before transport); and restrict prophylactic use to cases where the risk of disease is clearly evident. Remember to tell clients how to correctly administer antimicrobials to their animals. It is vital that you abide by responsible use guidelines or recommendations. Responsible use is an integral part of your professional code of conduct."
5. **Avoid off label use whenever possible:**
   "Using antimicrobials off label can lead to risks and side effects for animals. That's why it should be avoided wherever possible, and always supervised by a veterinarian."
6. **Be prepared to report your prescription data to the national Competent Authorities:**
   "Authorities need to track prescription data to effectively evaluate antimicrobial use and resistance development. When asked, be prepared to report your prescription data."
7. **Report any adverse effects due to antimicrobials use:**
   "Antimicrobials are essential for the treatment and prevention of infectious and zoonotic diseases in both animals and humans. Every use increases the risk of resistance developing. Everybody is affected and responsible for working to keep antimicrobials effective. You can play your part by making sure you report adverse effects antimicrobials cause, including if the treatment fails."

8. **More research and new products are necessary:**
"Research should be strongly encouraged to develop and make rapid diagnostic tests and sensitivity tests available – particularly ones that veterinarians can use on farms/in the field. A reliable regulatory environment is essential to promote the development of new antimicrobial products and alternatives to antimicrobials."

Conclusion

The veterinary surgeon has the ultimate responsibility for prescribing antimicrobials and in doing so should follow the concept of best veterinary practice. The responsibility of treating animals should be real, imparted by the owner and not merely nominal. That is to say, the veterinary surgeon must have good first-hand knowledge of the disease status of the herd and of the management procedures. Regular visits allow continuous appraisal and monitoring and the development of specific veterinary health plans that will define medication protocols.

The farm-to-fork principle must apply and pig producers should be aware that they are producing food, not pigs, and therefore antimicrobials must be used in the most responsible manner possible. Perhaps more importantly, high standards of biosecurity and hygiene must be maintained to reduce the need to use antimicrobials in the first place.

The global transmission of resistant bacteria has increased with the advent of widespread international travel and the cross-border trade in food and animals. The epidemiology of resistance is undoubtedly highly complex and may not be fully understood in the foreseeable future.

It is difficult to forecast trends in future use. Pig numbers are currently declining in the EU and a greater number of vaccines are becoming more widely available against the viral initiators of respiratory disease. Producers are becoming more geared up to administer water soluble medication and there is a desire to rely less on feed medication. With better health planning and greater use of vaccines, it is possible to obtain a decline in antimicrobial use. Certainly, the concept of treating pigs individually rather than the herd as a whole and focusing on the use of injectable treatments is in line with these trends.

Table 1. Critical categories of veterinary antimicrobials. Report of the 3rd meeting of the WHO advisory group, World Health Organization, 2012.

Critically important	Highly important	Important
Aminoglycosides (HC)	Rifamycins (HC)	Amynocyclitols (e.g. spectinomycin)
Cephalosporins (HC 3rd/4th)	Fosfomycin (HC)	Bicyclomycin
Macrolides (HC)	Ionophores	Fusidic acid
Penicillins (HC)	Lincosamides (HH)	Novobiocin
Phenicols (HH)	Pleuromutilins (HH)	Orthosomycins
Fluoroquinolones (HC)	Polypeptides (e.g. colistin sulphate) (HC)	Quinoxalines
Sulphonamides (HH)	-	Streptogramins
Tetracyclines (HH)	-	

HC = human critical; HH = Human highly important.

Table 2. Major presentations of antibiotics used in pig production.

Antimicrobial class	Premix	Water	Injection
Aminoglycosides and Amynocyclitols	Apramycin Spectinomycin (+ Lincomycin) Neomycin	Apramycin Spectinomycin (+ Lincomycin)	Streptomycin (+ Penicillin G)
Cephalosporins	-	-	Ceftiofur (G3) Cefquinome (G4)
Fluoroquinolones	-	Enrofloxacin (in some species)	Danofloxacin Enrofloxacin Marbofloxaicn
Lincosamides	Lincomycin (+ Spectinomycin)	Lincomycin (+ Spectinomycin)	Lincomycin
Macrolides	Tylosin Tylvalosin Tilmicosin	Tylosin Tylvalosin Tilmicosin	Tylosin Tildipirosin Tulathromycin
Penicillins	Phenoxymethyl penicillin (V) Amoxicillin (HC)	Phenoxymethyl penicillin (V) Amoxicillin	Procaine penicillin (G) Amoxicillin Ampicillin
Pleuromutilins	Tiamulin Valnemulin	Tiamulin	Tiamulin
Polymyxin	Colistin	Colistin	-
Sulphonamides	+ Trimethoprim	+ Trimethoprim	+ Trimethoprim
Tetracyclines	Oxytetracycline Chlortetracycline Doxycycline	Oxytetracycline Chlortetracycline Tetracycline Doxycycline	Oxytetracycline Doxycycline
Phenicols	Florfenicol	Florfenicol	Florfenicol

Common antimicrobial combinations are described between brackets.

Table 3. Mechanism of action and common resistance mechanisms of antimicrobial families.

Antimicrobial family	Subfamilies/Molecules	Mechanism of action	Resistance mechanisms
Β-lactam antibiotics	**Penicillin** Penicillin G, penicillin V, methicillin, oxacillin, ampicillin, amoxicillin, piperacillin **Cephalosporins** 1st to 2nd generation: cephalexin, cefradine, etc. 3rd to 4th generation: ceftiofur, cefquinome, cefixime, ceftazidime (use in human medicine) **Monobactams** Aztreonam **Carbapenems** Imipenem, meropenem	Inhibit cell wall synthesis. Bind to enzymes (PBPs) that help in the formation of peptidoglycans.	Primary production of β-lactamases (*bla* genes). Changes in the enzymes of the cell wall that prevent PBPs. *MecA* gene for resistance to methicillin (*Staphylococcus aureus*). Genes for production of β-lactamases (*bla*) TEM-1, TEM-2 and SHV-1, normally transferred by plasmids. Cephalosporinases Extended-spectrum β-lactamases (ESBL). CTX-M β-lactamase genes (*bla*) normally transferred by plasmids (extended-spectrum cephalosporins, ESC).
	Inhibitors of β-lactamases Clavulanic acid, sulbactam, tazobactam	Inhibit / bind to beta-lactam enzymes.	Resistance inhibition genes: cephalosporinase AmpC gene (bla_{cmy} subgroup), metalloenzyme genes. The mecA gene cannot bind to PBPs.
Polymyxins	Colistin	Action on the cell membrane: modify permeability.	Unclear: reduced bacterial permeability.
Tetracyclines	Chlortetracycline, oxytetracycline, doxycycline, minocycline	rRNA: bind to the 30S subunit of the ribosomes and interfere with the transfer of amino acids. Prevent the synthesis of proteins.	Efflux induced in *Escherichia coli*, etc. (*tetA*, *tetB*, *tetC* genes). Changes in the binding sites (*tetO* and *tetM* genes). Changes in the tetracycline molecule (rare).
Aminoglycosides Amynocyclitol	Streptomycin, neomycin, kanamycin, apramycin, gentamicin, amikacin Spectinomycin	rRNA: bind to the 30S subunit of the ribosomes and cause failures in the reading of the genetic code. Prevent the synthesis of proteins. Effect on the permeability of the cell wall.	The phosphorylation, adenilation and acetylation of aminoglycosides (*aph*, *aad* and *aac* genes) stop their binding. Streptomycin: only site of binding. Others: multiple binding sites, slow resistances, essentially by plasmids.

Table 3. Mechanism of action and common resistance mechanisms of antimicrobial families. Continuation.

Antimicrobial family	Subfamilies/Molecules	Mechanism of action	Resistance mechanisms
Macrolides/azalides (M)	Tilosyn, tylvalosin, tilmicosin, tulathromycin, azithromycin, erythromycin	rRna: bind to the 50S subunit of the ribosomes. Inhibit transpeptidation. Prevent protein synthesis.	The methylation of rRNA in gram bacteria (+) (*ermA*, *ermB*, *ermC* genes) inhibits their binding. Possible co-resistance (*misB* gene). Active efflux (*mef* gene). Possible enzymatic inactivation.
Lincosamides (L)	Lincomycin, clindamycin	rRna: bind to the 50S subunit of the ribosomes. Inhibit peptidyl transferase. Prevent protein synthesis.	The methylation of the 23S subunit of rRNA prevents their binding. Possible co-resistance (*misB* gene). Possible inactivation of the drug.
Streptogramins (S)	Virginiamycin	rRna: bind to the 50S subunit of the ribosomes. Prevent protein (class A and B) synthesis.	Methylation of rRNA in gram bacteria (+). Class A: activates efflux and inactivation of the drug (*vgA*, *vgaC* and *msrA*). Co-resistance with S, M, L and P. Class B: methylation of the 23S subunit of rRNA (*erm* genes).
Pleuromutilins (P)	Tiamulin, valnemulin	rRNA: bind to the 50S subunit of the ribosomes. Inhibit peptidyl transferase. Prevent the production of proteins.	Chromosomal mutations (chained). rRna methylation in Gram bacteria (+). Co-resistance genes (*vgA* y *vgaC*).
Phenicols	Thiamphenicol, florfenicol	Rrna: irreversibly bind to the 50S subunit of the ribosomes. Inhibit peptidyl transferase. Prevent the production of proteins.	The acetylation of the drug in enterobacteria (*catA* gene) prevents them from binding to the drug. Transmission through plasmids. Efflux (*cmlA* and *floR* genes); mutations in the "target" site and increase in barrier permeability.
Sulphonamides	Sulfadiazine	Purine synthesis for DNA. Interfere in folic acid synthesis.	Chromosomal mutations, but the resistance by plasmids and integrons is more common. Unblocking of the metabolic pathway by resistant dihydropteroate synthetase (*sul1*, *sul2* and *sul3* genes).

Table 3. Mechanism of action and common resistance mechanisms of antimicrobial families. Continuation.

Antimicrobial family	Subfamilies/Molecules	Mechanism of action	Resistance mechanisms
Diaminopyrimidins	Trimethoprim, ormetoprim	Purine synthesis for DNA. Interfere in folic acid synthesis.	Unblocking of the metabolic pathway by resistant dihydrofolate reductase (*dfr* gene). Often by transposons or integrons in the plasmids or chromosomes.
Quinolones and fluoroquinolones	**Quinolones** Nalidixic acid, oxolinic acid **Fluoroquinolones** flumequine, norfloxacin, enrofloxacin, ciprofloxacin, marbofloxacin	Interrupt the unwinding and rewinding of DNA by binding to the DNA gyrase or topoisomerase II (GyrA and GyrB subunits), topoisomerase IV (ParC and ParE subunits).	Modification of the "aim": DNA gyrase (*gyrA* and *gyrB* genes) resistance in a specific step + *parC* and *parE* genes (complete resistance). Resistance to nalidixic acid: only by mutation in the *gyrA* gene. Decrease in permeability: mutations in the external membrane porines (*ompF* gene). Efflux pumps. In principle, clonal resistance, but a plasmid gene (*qnr*) or integron has been discovered. Only *Campylobacter* spp. has type II topoisomerase, so there can be resistance in a specific step.

Table 4. Control points to decrease the spread of antimicrobial resistance in animals and humans.

Factors under the control of veterinary surgeons and farmers	Factors under control of food processors and people preparing and cooking food	Chance effects that may be influenced by lifestyle, environment, etc.	Factors under the control of physicians and their patients
Decision to use antimicrobials	Accuracy of documentation	Environment	Decision
Choice of antimicrobial	Accuracy of pig identification	Lifestyle	Choice of antimicrobial
Dose and route of administration	Routine and random sampling	Travel	Dose and route of administration
Duration of treatment	Abattoir hygiene	-	
Maintenance of accurate records	Meat transport and storage hygiene	-	
Observation of withholding times	Culinary hygiene and adequate cooking	-	
Farm hygiene	-	-	
Quality assurance	-	-	-

7 References

References

All the bibliographic references used in this book are listed in this chapter. Other noteworthy references not directly used in this book but that may be of interest to the readers have also been included.

1. Adamson, P. J., Wilson, W. D., Hirsh, D. C., Baggot, J. D. and Martin, L.D. Susceptibility of equine bacterial isolates to antimicrobial agents. *American Journal of Veterinary Research*, 46 (2): 447–450, 1985.
2. Aarestrup, F. M., Oliver Duran, C. and Burch, D. G. Antimicrobial resistance in swine production. *Animal Health Reviews*, 9 (2): 135–48, 2008.
3. Ageros, H., Friis, C. and Haugegaard, J. Water medication of a swine herd with amoxicilin. *Journal of Veterinary Pharmacology and Therapeutics*, 21: 199–202, 1998.
4. Alexander, T. J. L., Thornton, K., Boon, G., Lysons, R. J. and Gush, A. F. Medicated early weaning to obtain pigs free from pathogens endemic in the herd of origin. *Veterinary Record*, 106: 114–119, 1980.
5. Alexander, T. Zoonoses. *Proceedings 15th IPVS Congress*. Birmingham, England, 5-9 Jul. Vol 1. 167–173, 1998.
6. Alibaldi, F. S. and Lees, P. Antibiotic treatment for animals: Effect on bacterial population and dosage regimen optimisation. *International Journal of Antimicrobial Agents*, 14: 307–313, 2000.
7. Allaker, R. P., Lloyd, D. H. and Lamport, A. I. Bacterial interference in the control of exudative epidermitis of pigs. In: Von Tscharner, C. and Halliwell R. E. W. (eds). *Advances in Veterinary Dermatology*, vol. 1. London: Bailliere Tindall; 327–334, 1990.
8. Andersson, D. I. and Hughes, D. Persistence of antibiotic resistance in bacterial populations. *FEMS Microbiological Reviews*, 35 (5): 901–11, 2011.
9. Andresen, L. O., Ahrens, P., Daugaard, L. and Bille-Hansen, V. Exudative epidermitis in pigs caused by toxigenic *Staphylococcus chromogenes*. *Veterinary Microbiology*, 105: 291–300, 2005.
10. Andrews, J. J., Lucas, T. E. and Johnson, D. D. Prevention and control of experimentally induced *Pasteurella multocida* pneumonia in swine by the use of chlortetracycline administered in feed. *Agri-practice*, 9: 33–38.1998.
11. Apley, M. An antimicrobial targeting toolbox for the swine practitioner. *Allen D. Leman Swine Conference*, 76–83, 2005.
12. Aramayona, J. J., Mora, J., Fraile, L. J., Abadía, A. R., García, M. A. and Bregante, M. A. Penetration of enrofloxacin and ciprofloxacin into breast milk and pharmacokinetics of the drugs in lactating rabbits and neonatal offspring. *American Journal of Veterinary Research*, 57 (4): 547–553, 1996.
13. Armstrong, C. H., Hooper, B. E. and Martin, C. E. Microflora associated with agalactia syndrome in sows. *American Journal of Veterinary Research*, 29: 1401–1407, 1968.
14. Awad Masalmeh, M., Baumgartner, W., Passering, A., Silber, R. and Hinterdorfer, F. Bakteriologische Untersuchungen bei an puerperaler Mastitis (MMA-Syndrom) erkrankten Sauen verschiedener Tierbestände Österreichs (Bacteriological studies in sows with puerperal mastitis in different herds in Austria). *Tierärztl Umsch*, 45: 526–535, 1990.
15. Bäckström, L. Environment and animal health in piglet production. *Acta Veterinaria Scandinavica*, Suppl. 41: 1–240, 1973.
16. Bäckström, L. A. C., Morkoc, J., Connor, R. and Price, W. Clinical study of mastitis–metritis–agalactia in sows in Illinois. *Journal of the American Veterinary Medical Association*, 185: 70–73, 1984.
17. Baekbo, P., Madsen, K. S., Aagard, M. and Szancer, J. Eradication of *Mycoplasma*

hyopneumoniae from infected herds without restocking. *Proceedings 13th International Pig Veterinary Society Congress*, Bangkok, Thailand, p. 135, 1994.

18. Baer, C. and Bilkei, G. Ultrasonographic and gross pathological findings in the mammary glands of weaned sows having suffered recidiving mastitis metritis agalactia. *Reproduction in Domestic Animals*, 40 (6): 544–547, 2005.

19. Baggot, J. D. *The physiological basis of veterinary clinical pharmacology*. Blackwell Science Ltd, Oxford, 2001.

20. Baldwin, D. R., Honeybourne, D. and Wise, R. Pulmonary disposition of antimicrobial agents: In vivo observations and clinical relevance. *Antimicrobial Agents Chemotherapy*, 36: 1176–1180, 1992.

21. Berner, H. Importance of urinary tract infections in development of puerperal endometritis in the sow. *Tierärzt Umsch*, 39: 450–458, 1984.

22. Berner, H. Cystitis in the diagnosis of metritis-mastitis-agalactia. *Prakt Tierarzt*, 69: 124–130, 1988.

23. Bertschinger, H. U. and Bühlmann, A. Absence of protective immunity in mammary glands after experimentally induced coliform mastitis. *Proceeedings 11th International Pig Veterinary Society Congress*, Lausanne, Switzerland, p. 175, 1990.

24. Bertschinger, H. U. Postweaning *Escherichia coli* diarrhea and edema disease. In: Straw B. E., D'Allaire, S., Mengeling, W. L. and Taylor D. J. (eds.) *Diseases of Swine*. Ames, Iowa: Iowa States University Press, pp. 441–454, 1999.

25. Bertschinger, H. U. Coliform Mastitis. In: Straw B. E., D'Allaire S., Mengeling W. L., Taylor D. J. (eds.). *Diseases of Swine*. Ames: Iowa State University Press, pp. 457–464, 1999.

26. Bhullar, K., Waglechner, N., Pawlowski, A., Koteva, K., Banks, E. D, Johnston, M. D., Barton, H.A. and Wright, G. D. Antibiotic resistance is prevalent in an isolated cave microbiome. *PLoS One*, 7 (4): e34953, doi: 10.1371/journal.pone.0034953. Epub 2012 Apr 11.

27. Blaha, T., Erler, W. and Burch, D. G. Swine dysentery control in the German Democratic Republic and the suitability of tiamulin injections in the programme. *Veterinary Record*, 121: 416, 1987.

28. Blondeau, J. M., Zhao, X., Hanson, G. and Drlica, K. Mutant prevention concentrations of fluorquinolones for clinical isolates of *Streptococcus pneumoniae. Antimicrobial Agents Chemotherapy*, 45: 433–438, 2001.

29. Blood, D. C. and Radostits, O. M. *Medicina Veterinaria*. Editorial Interamericana-McGraw-Hill, Madrid, 1992.

30. Bloom, P. B. and Rosser, E. J. Efficacy of once-daily clindamycin hydrochloride in the treatment of superficial bacterial pyoderma in dogs. *Journal of the American Hospital Association*, 37: 537–542, 2001.

31. Bodor, N. and Brewster, M. E. Problems of delivery of drugs to the brain. *Pharmacological Therapy*, 19: 337–386, 1982.

32. Bond, R. Therapy of canine pyoderma. *20th Annual Congress of the ESVD-ECVD*. Chalkidiki, Grecia, 2005.

33. Bostedt, H., Maier, G., Herfen, K. and Hospen, R. Clinical examinations on gilts with puerperal septicaemia and toxaemia. *Tierarztl Prax Ausg G Grosstiere Nutztiere*, 26 (6): 332–338, 1998.

34. Bousquet, E., Pommier, P., Wessel-Robert, S., Morvan, H., Benoit-Valiergue, H. and Laval, A. Efficacy of doxycycline in feed for the control of pneumonia caused by *Pasteurella multocida* and *Mycoplasma hyopneumoniae* in fattening pigs. *Veterinary Record*, 143 (10): 269–72, 1998.

35. Bramley, A. J. and Dodd, F.H. Reviews of the progress of dairy siences: Mastitis control progress and prospects. *Journal of Dairy Science*, 51: 481–512, 1984.

36. Bretzlaff, K. N. Rationale for treatment of endometritis in the dairy cow. *Veterinary Clinics of North America: Food Animal Practice*, 3: 593–607, 1987.

37. Brown, D. and Cantón, R. Bases for clinical categorization. In: Coruvalin, P., Leclerq, R. and Rice, L. B. (eds.), *Antibiogram*, pp. 37–45. Eska Publishing ASM Press, Portland, OR, 2010.

38. Brunton, L., Lazo, J. and Parker, K. *Goodman & Gilman's. The Pharmacological Basis of Therapeutics*, 11th ed. McGraw-Hill education, 2006.

39. Burch, D. G. S. Pharmacokinetics, minimal inhibitory concentrations and efficacy model relationships for some gut infections in pigs. *The Pig Journal*, 52: 48–61, 2003.

40. Burch, D. G. S. Pharmacokinetic, pharmacodynamic and clinical correlations relating to the therapy of colonic infections in the pig and breakpoint determinations. *The Pig Journal*, 56: 8–24, 2005a.

41. Burch, D. G. S. Pharmacokinetic, pharmacodynamic and clinical correlations relating to the therapy of *Lawsonia intracellularis* infections, the cause of porcine proliferative enteropathy ('ileitis') in the pig. *The Pig Journal*, 56: 25–44, 2005b.

42. Burch, D. G. S. Mycoplasma *eradication. The Danish way.* Pig World, 2006. www.octagon-services.co.uk/articles/eradication.htm.

43. Burch, D. G. S. Pharmacokinetics of antimicrobials at different levels of the intestinal tract and their relationship to *Escherichia coli* resistance patterns in the pig. *The Pig Journal*, 59: 91–111, 2007.

44. Burch, D. G. S., Duran, C. O. and Aarestrup, F. M. Guidelines for antimicrobial use in swine. In: Guardabassi L., Jensen L. B. andKruse H. (eds), *Guide to Antimicrobial Use in Animals*. Oxford: Wiley Blackwell; 122–123, 2008.

45. Burch, D. G. S. *Examination of the pharmacokinetic/pharmacodynamic (PK/PD) relationships of orally administered antimicrobials and their correlation with the therapy of various bacterial and mycoplasmal infections in pigs*. Fellowship Thesis. Royal College of Veterinary Surgeons. 2012.

46. Burrows, M. R., Morgan, J. H., Tasker, J. B. and Martin, M. In-feed Aivlosin for control of experimental enzootic pneumonia in pigs. *Proceedings 17th International Pig Veterinary Society Congress*, Ames, Iowa, USA, 2, p. 141, 2002.

47. Cameron R. Diseases of the skin. In: Straw B. E., Zimmerman J. J., D'Allaire S. et al. (eds.). *Diseases of Swine*, 9th ed. Ames, IA: Blackwell Publishing. pp. 179–198, 2006.

48. Cantón, R., Coque, T. M. and Baquero, F. Multi-resistant Gram-negative bacilli: From epidemics to endemics. *Current Opinion Infectious Disease*, 16: 315–325, *2003*.

49. Cantón, R. and Morosini, M. I. Emergence and spread of antibiotic resistance following exposure to antibiotics. *FEMS Microbiology Reviews*, 35 (5): 977–91, 2011.

50. Carvajal, A., De Arriba, M. L., Rodríguez, H., Vidal, A. B., Duhamel, G. E. and Rubio, P. Prevalence of Brachyspira species in pigs with diarrhoea in Spain. *Veterinary Record*, 158: 700–701, 2006.

51. Casteel, S. W., Brown, L. D., Lattimer, J. and Dunsmore, M. Fasting and Feeding Effects on Gastric Emptying Time in Juvenile Swine. *Contemporary Top Laboratory Animal Science*, 37 (5): 106–108, 1998.

52. Cerne, F. and Jochle, W. Clinical evaluations of a new prostaglandin analog in pigs: 1. Control of parturition and of the MMA-syndrome. *Theriogenology*, 16: 459–467, 1981.

53. Chen, S., Wang, Y., Chen, F., Yang, H., Gan, M. and Zheng, S. J. A highly pathogenic strain of *Staphylococcus sciuri* caused fatal exudative epidermitis in piglets. *PLoS One*, 2 (1): e147, 2007.

54. Clemens, E. T., Stevens, C. E. and Southworth, M. Sites of organic acid production and pattern of digesta movement in the gastrointestinal tract of swine. *Journal of Nutrition*, 105: 759–768, 1975.

55. CLSI 2011. Performance standards for antimicrobial susceptibility testing. *Twenty-first informational supplement. M100 - S21*, Vol. 31, nº 1.2011 clsi.pdf, 2011.

56. Constable, P. D. and Morin, D.E. Treatment of clinical mastitis using antimicrobial

susceptibility profiles for treatment decisions. *Veterinary Clinics of North America: Food Animal Practice,* 19: 139–155, 2003.

57. Constable, P. D. Antimicrobial use in the treatment of calf diarrhoea. *Journal of Veterinary Internal Medicine,* 18: 8–17, 2004.

58. Conte, J. E., Golden, J., Duncan, S., McKenna, E., Lin, E. and Zurlinden, E. Single-dose intrapulmonary pharmacokinetics of azithromycin, clarithromycin, ciprofloxacin, and cefuroxime in volunteer subjects. *Antimicrobial Agents and Chemotherapy,* 40: 1617–1622, 1996.

59. Christensen, G., Sorensen, V., Mousing, J. Diseases of the respiratory system. In: *Disease of Swine*, 8th ed. Edited by Straw, B. A, D'Allaire, S., Mengeling, W. L. and Taylor, D. J. Iowa State University Press, Ames, Iowa, 1999.

60. Craig, W. A. and Ebert, S. C. Protein binding and its significance in antibacterial therapy. *Infectious Disease Clinics North America.* 3 (3): 407–414, 1989.

61. Craig, W. A. and Andes, W. Pharmacokinetics and pharmacodynamic of antibiotics in otitis media. *Pediatric Infectious Disease Journal,* 15: 255–59, 1996.

62. Craig, W. A. Pharmacokinetic/pharmacodynamic parameters: Rationale for antibacterial dosing of mice and men. *Clinical infectious diseases*, 26: 1–12, 1998.

63. Craig, W. A. Proof of concept: Performance testing in models. *Clinical Microbiology and Infection,* 10 (Suppl. 2): 12–17, 2004.

64. Davis, S. S., Illum, L. and Hinchcliffe, M. Gastrointestinal transit of dosage forms in the pig. *Journal of Pharmacy and Pharmacology*, 53, 33–39, 2001.

65. D'Costa, V. M., King, C. E., Kalan, L., Morar, M., Sung, W. W., Schwarz, C., Froese, D., Zazula, G., Calmels, F., Debruyne, R., Golding, G. B., Poinar, H. N. and Wright, G. D. Antibiotic resistance is ancient. *Nature*, 477 (7365): 457–61, 2011.

66. Dee, S. A. The PRDC: Are subpopulations important? *Journal of Swine Health and Production*, 4; 3: 147–149, 1996.

67. De Lange, E. C. M. and Danhof, M. Considerations in the use of cerebrospinal fluid pharmacokinetics to predict brain target concentrations in the clinical setting: Implications of the barriers between blood and brain. *Clinical Pharmacokinetics,* 41: 691–703, 2002.

68. De Lange, E. C. M, Ravenstijn, P. G. M, Groenendaal, D. and Van Steeg, T. J. Towards the prediction of CNS Drug-effect profiles in physiological and pathological conditions using microdialysis ands mechanism-based pharmacokinetic-pharmacodynamic modelling. *The AAPS journal*, 7 (3): E532-E543, 2005.

69. De Boer, A. G., Van der Sandt, I. and Gaillard, P. J., The role of drug transporters at the blood-brain barrier. *Annual Review of Pharmacology and Toxicology*, 43: 629–656, 2003.

70. De Boer, D. J. Strategies for management of recurrent pyoderma in dogs. *Veterinary Clinics of North America: Small Animal Practice,* 20 (6): 1509–1524, 1990.

71. Del Castillo, J. R. E., Elsener, J. and Martineau, G. P. Pharmacokinetic modelling of in-feed tetracyclines in pigs using a meta-analysis compartmental approach. *Journal of Swine Health and Production*, 6 (5): 189–202, 1998.

72. Demanuelle, T. C., Ihrke, P. J., Brandt, C. M., Kass, P. H. and Vulliet, P. R. Determination of skin concentrations of enrofloxacin in dogs with pyoderma. *American Journal of Veterinary Research*, 59 (12): 1599–1604, 1998.

73. Desrosiers, R. and Martineau, G. P. Control and economical aspects of swine pleuropneumonia n fattening units. *Proceedings 8th IPVS*, Ghent, Belgium, 1984.

74. Desrosiers, R. Diagnosis and control of swine respiratory diseases. *Proceedings of the American Association of Swine Practitioners.* pp. 333–344, 1997.

75. Ding, H., Li, Y., Chen, Z., Rizwan-ul-Haq, M. and Zeng, Z. Plasma and tissue cage fluid pharmacokinetics of marbofloxacin after intravenous, intramuscular, and oral single-dose application in pigs. *Journal of Veterinary Pharmacology and Therapeutics*, 33 (5): 507–10, 2010.

76. Dowling, P. M. Antimicrobial therapy of skin and ear infections. *Canadian Veterinary Journal*, 37: 695–699, 1996.

77. Dowling, P. M. Antimicrobial therapy of urinary tract infections. *Canadian Veterinary Journal*, 37: 438–441, 1996.

78. Dowling, P. M. Clinical pharmacology of nervous system diseases. *Veterinary Clinics of North America: Equine Practice*, 15 (3): 575–588, 1999.

79. Drlica, K. A strategy for fighting antibiotic resistance. *ASM News*, 67: 27–33, 2001.

80. Drusano, G. L. Antimicrobial pharmacodynamics: Critical interactions of "bug and drug". *Nature reviews Microbiology*, 2: 289–300, 2004.

81. Drusano, G. L. Infection site concentrations: their therapeutic importance and the macrolide and macrolide-like class of antibiotics. *Pharmacotherapy*, 25: 150S–158S, 2005.

82. Dudley, M. N. Pharmacodynamics and pharmacokinetics of antibiotics with special reference to the fluorquinolones. *American Journal of Medicine*, 91 (6A): 45–50, 1991.

83. Duhamel, G., Cowan, T. R., *Proceedings of the American Association of Swine Practitioners*, Quebec City, Canada, pp. 225–229, 1997.

84. Ebert, S. C. and Craig, W. A. Pharmacodynamic properties of antibiotics: Application to drug monitoring and dosage regimen design. *Infection Control and Hospital Epidemiology*, 11: 319–226, 1990.

85. Ehinger, A. M. and Kietzmann, M. Tissue distribution of benzylpenicillin after intrammary administration in the isolated perfused bovine udder. *Journal of Veterinary Pharmacology and Therapeutics*, 23: 303–310, 2000.

86. Ensink, J. M., Klein, W. R., Barneveld, A., Vulto, A. G., Van Miert, A. S. and Tukker, J. J. Distribution of penicilins into subcutaneous tissue chambers in ponies. *Journal of Veterinary Pharmacology and Therapeutics*, 19 (6): 439–444, 1996.

87. Erskine, R., Kirk, J. H., Tyler, J. W. and Degraves, F. J. Advances in the therapy for mastitis. *Veterinary Clinics of North America: Food Animal Practice*, 9: 499–517, 1993.

88. Erskine, R., Wagner, S. and Degraves, F. J. Mastitis therapy and pharmacology. *Veterinary Clinics of North America: Food Animal Practice*, 19: 109–138, 2003.

89. European Committee on Antimicrobial Susceptibility Testing. *Breakpoint tables for interpretation of MICs and zone diameters. Version 1.3*. Available at http: //www.eucast.org [viewed 2011].

90. Fairbrother, J. M., Nadeau, E. and Gyles, C. L. *Escherichia coli* in postweaning diarrhoea in pigs: an update on bacterial types, pathogenesis, and prevention strategies. *Animal Health Research Reviews*, 6 (1): 17–39, 2005.

91. Florea, N. F and Nightingale, C. H. Review of the pharmacodynamics of antibiotic use in animal food production. *Diagnostic Microbiology and Infectious Disease*, 49: 105–108, 2004.

92. Forrest, A., Nix, D., Ballow, D. E., Goss, C. H., Birmingham, M. C. and Schentag, J. J. Pharmacodynamics of IV ciprofloxacin in seriously ill patients. *Antimicrobial agents and Chemotherapy*, 37: 1073–1081, 1993.

93. Forrest, A. Patient studies modeling Surrogates and their Linkages: MICs, clinical Scoring, and PK/PD indices of effect. *15th ISAP International Symposium Surrogate Markers in the development of Anti-infectives. A post-ICAAC 2005 meeting*, Washington, DC. December 19th, 2005.

94. Fraile, L. J., Aramayona, J. J., García, M. A., Abadía, A. R. and Bregante, M. A. Administración de fármacos a pacientes pediátricos. *Medicina Veterinaria*, 11 (6): 325–331, 1994.

95. Fraile, L. J., Aramayona, J. J., García, M. A., Abadía, A. R. and Bregante, M. A. Uso de aminoglucósidos durante el período perinatal. *Medicina Veterinaria,* 12 (10): 621–629, 1995.

96. Fraile L., Alegre, A., López-Jiménez, R., Nofrarías, M. and Segalés, J. Risk factors associated with pleuritis and cranio-ventral pulmonary consolidation in slaughter-aged pigs. *Veterinary Journal,* 184 (3): 326–33, 2010.

97. Frimodt-Moller, N. How predictive is PK/PD for antibacterial agents? *International Journal of Antimicrobial Agents*, 19: 333–339, 2002a.

98. Frimodt-Moller, N. Correlation between pharmacokinetic/pharmacodynamic parameters and efficacy for antibiotics in the treatment of urinary tract infection. *International Journal of Antimicrobial Agents*, 19: 546–553, 2002b.

99. Friis, C. *The role of pharmacokinetics and pharmacodynamics in the treatment of infectious diseases*. Belgium, 2004. Personal communication.

100. Furniss S. J. Measurement of rectal temperature to predict mastitis, metritis and agalactia (MMA) in sows after farrowing. *Preventive Veterinary Medicine*, 5: 133–139, 1987.

101. Futagawa-Saito, K., Ba-Thein, W. and Fukuyasu, T. Antimicrobial susceptibilities of exfoliative toxigenic and non-toxigenic *Staphylococcus hyicus* strains in Japan. *Journal of Veterinary Medical Science*, 71 (5): 681–4, 2009.

102. FVE, Federation of Veterinarians of Europe. *Antibiotic Resistance and Prudent use of Antibiotics in Veterinary Medicine*, 1999 (http: //www.fve.org/papers/pdf/vetmed/position_papers/antibioen.pdf).

103. Gall, S., Hemsell, D. L., McGregor, J. A., Martens, M. G., Pitkin, D. and Allen, S. Tissue penetration of meropenem in patients undergoing gynecologic surgery. *Clinical Infectious Diseases*, Suppl 2: S178–80, 1997.

104. Ganiere, J. P., Medaille, C. and Mangion, C. Antimicrobial activity of *Staphylococcus intermedius* clinical isolates from canine pyoderma. *Journal of Veterinary Medicine B*, 52: 25–31, 2005.

105. Ganiere, J. P., Medaille, C., Limet, A, Ruvoen, N. and Andre-Fontaine, G. Antimicrobial activity of enrofloxacin against *Staphylococcus intermedius* strains isolated from canine pyodermas. *Veterinary dermatology*, 12: 171–175, 2001.

106. García-Castillo, M., Del Campo, R., Baquero, F., Morosini, M. I., Turrientes, M. C., Zamora, J. and Cantón, R. Stationary biofilm growth normalizes mutation frequencies and mutant prevention concentrations in *Pseudomonas aeruginosa* from cystic fibrosis patients. *Clinical Microbiology Infection*, 17 (5): 704–11, 2011.

107. Gebhart, C. J. *Lawsonia intracellularis*: Overview and research update. *First Novartis Animal Health European Swine Ileitis/Colitis Workshop*, Alpbach, Austria, 2004.

108. Gibaldi, M. and Perrier, D. *Farmacocinética*. Editorial Reverté, S.A. Barcelona, 1982.

109. Giesting, D. W. and Easte, R. A. Response of starter pigs to supplementation of corn soybean meal diets with organic acids. *Journal of Animal Science,* 60: 1288–1294, 1985.

110. Göransson, L. The effect of feed allowance in late pregnancy on the occurrence of agalactia post partum in the sow. *Journal of Veterinary Medicine A*, 36: 505–513, 1989.

111. Gottschalk, M. and Segura, M. The pathogenesis of the meningitis caused by *Streptococcus suis*: The unresolved questions. *Veterinary Microbiology*, 76: 259–272, 2000.

112. Gottschalk, M., Xu, J., Calzas, C. and Segura, M. *Streptococcus suis*: a new emerging or an old neglected zoonotic pathogen? *Future Microbiology,* 5 (3): 371–391, 2010.

113. Gottschalk, M. *Streptococcosis*. In: *Diseases of Swine*. Karriker L., Ramirez A., Schwartz

K.J., Stevenson G., Zimmerman J. (eds). Wiley Publishers, NJ, USA, 2011.

114. Gruet, P., Maincent, P., Berthelot, X. and Kaltsatos, K. Bovine mastitis and intrammary drug delivery: Review and perspectives. *Advanced drug Delivery Reviews*, 50: 245–259, 2001.

115. Giguère, S., Huang, R., Malinski, T. J., Dorr, P. M., Tessman, R. K. and Somerville, B. A. Disposition of gamithromycin in plasma, pulmonary epithelial lining fluid, bronchoalveolar cells, and lung tissue in cattle. *American Journal of Veterinary Research*. 72 (3): 326–330, 2011.

116. Gutiérrez-Martín, C. B., Del Blanco N. G., Blanco, M., Navas, J. and Rodríguez-Ferri, E. F. Changes in antimicrobial susceptibility of *Actinobacillus pleuropneumoniae* isolated from pigs in Spain during the last decade. *Veterinary Microbiology*, 115 (1 – 3): 218–22, 2006.

117. Guyonnet, J., Monnoyer, S., Manco, B. Alibaldi, F.S. and Lees, P. In vivo pharmacokinetics and in vitro pharmacodynamics as a basis for predicting dosage of colistin in piglets gastrointestinal disease. *Journal of Veterinary Pharmacology and Therapeutics*, 26 (suppl 1): 148–149, 2003.

118. Guyton, A. C. and Hall, J. E. *Human physiology and mechanisms of disease*. Saunders (W.B.) Co Ltd, 1996.

119. Halgaard, C. Epidemiologic factors in puerperal diseases of sow. *Nord Veterinary Medicine*, 35 (4): 161–174, 1983.

120. Hampson, D. J., Fellstrom, C. and Thomson, J. R. Swine dysentery. In: Straw, B. E., Zimmerman, J. J., D'Allaire, S. et al. (eds.), *Diseases of Swine*, 9th ed. Blackwell Publishing Professional, Ames, IA, USA, pp. 785–805, 2006.

121. Hannan, P. C. T., Bhogal, B. S. and Fish, J. P. Tylosin tartrate and tiamulin effects on experimental piglet pneumonia induced with pneumonic pig lung homogenate containing mycoplasmas, bacteria and viruses. *Research in Veterinary Science*, 33: 76–88, 1982.

122. Hannan, P. C. T., Windsor, H. M. and Ripley, P. H. In vitro susceptibilities of recent field isolates of *Mycoplasma hyopneumoniae* and *Mycoplasma hyosynoviae* to valnemulin (Econor), tiamulin and enrofloxacin and the in vitro development of resistance to certain antimicrobial agents in *Mycoplasma hyopneumoniae*. *Research in Veterinary Science*, 63 (2): 157–60, 1997.

123. Hannan, P. C. T. Guidelines and recommendations for antimicrobial minimum inhibitory concentration (MIC) testing against veterinary mycoplasma species. *Veterinary Research*, 31: 373–395, 2000.

124. Heinritzi, K. and Hagn, J. Untersuchungen zur Wirksamkeit und Verträglichkeit des neu entwickelten Cephalosporins Cefquinom bei an puerperaler Septikämie und Toxämie erkrankten Sauen (Comparison of therapeutic performance of the new Cephalosporin Cefquinome with other treatment regimes in gilts with puerperal septicaemia and toxaemia syndrome) *Tierärztl Prax*, 27: 114–121, 1999.

125. Henry, S. C. and Apley, M. Therapeutics. In *Disease of Swine*, 8th ed, Straw, B. A, D'Allaire, S., Mengeling, W. L. and Taylor, D. J. (eds.). Iowa State University Press, Ames, Iowa, 1999.

126. Hidalgo, A., Carvajal, A., Vester, B., Pringle, M., Naharro, G. and Rubio, P. Trends towards lower antimicrobial susceptibility and characterization of acquired resistance among clinical isolates of *Brachyspira hyodysenteriae* in Spain. *Antimicrobial Agents and Chemotherapy*, 55 (7): 3330–7, 2011.

127. Hirsch, A. C., Philipp, H. and Kleemann, R. Investigation on the efficacy of meloxicam in sows with mastitis-metritis-agalactia syndrome. *Journal of Veterinary Pharmacology and Therapeutics*, 26: 355–360, 2003.

128. Høiby, N., Bjarnsholt, T., Givskov, M., Molin, S. and Ciofu, O. Antibiotic resistance

of bacterial biofilms. *International Journal of Antimicrobial Agents*, 35 (4): 322–32, 2010.

129. Holm, A. and Poulsen H. D. Swine nutrition management update: zinc oxide in treating *E. coli* diarrhea in pigs after weaning. *Compendium on Continuing Education for the Practicing Veterinarian,* 18: S26–S48, 1996.

130. Holtz, W., Hartmann, J. F. and Welp, C. Induction of parturition in swine with prostaglandin analogs and oxytocin. *Theriogenology*, 19: 583–592, 1983.

131. Homma, T., Hori, T., Sugimori, G. and Yamano, Y. Pharmacodynamic assessment based on mutant prevention concentrations of fluoroquinolones to prevent the emergence of resistant mutants of *Streptococcus pneumoniae. Antimicrobial Agents and Chemotherapy*, 51: 3810–3815, 2007.

132. Hoover, T. *Porcine Respiratory Disease Complex*. Pfizer Animal Health. Technical Bulletin. October 1996.

133. Horspool, L. J. I. Van Laar, P. V., Van Den Bos, R. and Manwhinney, I. Treatment of canine pyoderma with ibafloxacin and marbofloxacin-fluorquinolones with different pharmacokinetic profiles. *Journal of Veterinary Pharmacology and Therapeutics*, 27: 147–153, 2004.

134. Hultén, F., Persson A., Eliasson-Selling L., Heldmer, E., Lindberg, M., Sjögren, U., Kugelberg, C. and Ehlorsson, C. J. Evaluation of environmental and management-related risk factors associated with chronic mastitis in sows. *American Journal of Veterinary Research*, 65: 1398–1403, 2004.

135. Hurd, H. S. Antibiotic use and public policy: The science and politics behind the current debate. *Pfizer Symposium*, Vancouver, 2010.

136. Hyatt, J. M., Luzier, A. B., Forrest, A., Ballow, C. H. and Schentag, J. J. Modelling the response of pneumonia to antimicrobial therapy. *Antimicrobial Agents and Chemotherapy*, 41 (6): 1269–1274, 1997.

137. Hybschmann, G. K., Ersboll, A. K., Vigre, H., Baadsgaard, N. P. and Houe, H. Herd-level risk factors for antimicrobial demanding gastrointestinal diseases in Danish herds with finisher pigs: a register-based study. *Preventive Veterinary Medicine*, 98 (2–3): 190–197, 2011.

138. Ihrke, P. J. Therapeutic strategies involving antimicrobial treatment of the skin in small animals. *Journal of the American Veterinary Medical Association*, 185 (10): 1165–1168, 1984.

139. Jacobs, M. R. How can we predict bacterial eradication? *International Journal of Infectious Disease*, 7: S13–S20, 2003.

140. Jacobson, M., Fellström, C. and Jensen-Waern, M. Porcine proliferative enteropathy: an important disease with questions remaining to be solved. *Veterinary Journal*, 184: 264–268, 2010.

141. Jensen, G. M., Lykkesfeld, J., Frydendahl, K., Moller, K. and Svendsen, O. Pharmacokinetics of amoxicillin after oral administration in recently weaned piglets with experimentally inducded *Escherichia coli* subtype 0149: F4 diarrhoea. *American Journal of Veterinary Research*, 65 (7): 992–995, 2004.

142. Jones, J. E. T. Bacterial mastitis and endometritis in sows. *Proceedings 4th International Pig Veterinary Society Congress*, Ames, USA, 4: E6, 1976.

143. Kahlmeter, G., Brown, D. F., Goldstein, F. W., MacGowan, A. P., Mouton, J. W., Osterlund A., Rodloff, A., Steinbakk, M., Urbaskova P. and Vatopoulos, A. European harmonization of MIC breakpoints for antimicrobial susceptibility testing of bacteria. *Journal of Antimicrobial Chemotherapy*, 52: 145–148, 2003.

144. Karlsson, M., Gunnarsson, A. and Franklin, A. Susceptibility to pleuromutilins in *Brachyspira (Serpulina) hyodysenteriae. Animal Health Research Review,* 2: 59–65, 2001.

145. Karlsson, M., Oxberry, S. L. and Hampson, D. J. Antimicrobial susceptibility testing of

Australian isolates of *Brachyspira hyodysenteriae* using a new broth dilution method. *Veterinary Microbiology*, 84: 123–133, 2002.

146. Karlsson, M., Fellstrom, C., Gunnarsson, A., Landen, A. and Franklin, A. Antimicrobial susceptibility testing of porcine *Brachyspira* (*Serpulina*) species isolates. *Journal of Clinical Microbiology*, 41: 2596–2604, 2003.

147. Kemper, N. and Gerjets, I. Bacteria in milk from anterior and posterior mammary glands in sows affected and unaffected by postpartum dysgalactia syndrome (PPDS). *Acta Veterinaria Scandinavica*, 51: 26, 2009

148. Kim, J. and Chae, C. Concurrent presence of porcine circovirus type 2 and porcine parvovirus in retrospective cases of exudative epidermitis in pigs. *Veterinary Journal*, 167 (1): 104–6, 2004.

149. Klopfenstein, C., Farmer, C., Martineau, G.P. Diseases of the mammary glands and lactation problems. In: Straw B. E. and Zimmermann J. J. and Taylor D. J. (eds), *Diseases of swine*, 4th ed. Iowa State University Press, pp. 833–860, 2006.

150. Kohanski, M. A., DePristo, M. A. and Collins, J. J. Sublethal antibiotic treatment leads to multidrug resistance via radical-induced mutagenesis. *Molecular Cell*, 37: 311–320, 2010.

151. Kubo, M., Yamamoto, K., Ibayashi, T. and DeKeyser, H. Study on the effect of feed medication with lincomycin against artificial infection of mycoplasmal pneumonia in swine. *Proceedings 11th International Pig Veterinary Society Congress*, Lausanne, Switzerland, p. 90, 1990.

152. La, T., Phillips, D. and Hampson, D. Develpoment of a duplex PCR assay for detection of *Brachyspira hyodysenteriae* and *Brachyspira pilosicoli* in pig feces. *Journal of Clinical Microbiology*, Vol 41, 3372–3375, 2003.

153. Larsen, I. and Thorup, F. The Diagnosis of MMA. *19th International Pig Veterinary Society Congress*, Copenhagen, Denmark. p. 256, 2006.

154. Lauritzen, B., Lykkesfeldt, J. and Friis, C. Evaluation of single dose versus a divided dose regimen of danofloxacin in treatment of *Actinobacillus pleuropneumoniae* infection in pigs. *Research in Veterinary Science*, 74: 271–277, 2003.

155. Lees, P. and Alibaldi, F. Rationalising dosage regimens of antimicrobial drugs: A pharmacological perspective. *Journal Medical Microbiology*, 49 (11): 943–945, 2000.

156. Lees, P. Rational dosing: animals versus humans. *8th ISAP Symposium Developments in Pharmacokinetics and Pharmacodynamics (PK/PD): optimizing efficacy and prevention of resistance*, Nijmegen, The Netherlands, 4–6 July 2001.

157. Lees, P. and Alibaldi, F. Principios de antibioterapia. In: *Farmacología y terapéutica veterinaria*, Botana L. M, Landoni F., Martín-Jiménez, T. (eds). McGraw-Hill interamericana. 2002[a].

158. Lees, P. and Alibaldi, F. Rational dosing of antimicrobial drugs: animals versus humans. *International Journal of Antimicrobial Agents*, 19: 269–284, 2002[b].

159. Lees, P., Cunningham, F. M. and Elliott, J. Principles of pharmacodynamics and their application in veterinary pharmacology. *Journal of Veterinary Pharmacology and Therapeutics*, 27: 397–414, 2004[a].

160. Lees, P., Alibaldi, F. and Toutain, P. L. PK-PD Modelling: An alternative to dose titration studies for antimicrobial drug dose selection. *Journal of Regulatory Affairs*. 175–180, 2004[b].

161. Lees, P., Concordet, D., Alibaldi, F. and Toutain, P. L. Drug selection and optimization of dosage schedules to minimize antimicrobial resistance. Chapter five, in: *Antimicrobial resistance in bacteria of animal origin*, Aarestrup, F. M. (ed.), pp. 49–71, 2006.

162. Lefebvre, R. C. and Stock A. E. Therapeutic efficiency of antibiotics and prostaglandin

F2α in postpartum dairy cows with clinical endometritis: an evidence-based evaluation. *Veterinary Clinics of North America: Food Animal Practice*, 28 (1): 79–96, 2012.

163. Levy, S. Antibiotic resistance: an ecological imbalance. Antibiotic Resistance: Origins, Evolution, Selection and Spread. *Ciba Foundation Symposium*, 207, pp. 1–14, 1997.

164. Lewis, K. Persister cells. *Annual Review Microbiolog*, 64: 357–372, 2010.

165. Lin, J. H. Tissue distribution and pharmacodynamics: a complicated relationship. *Current Drug Metabolism*, 7 (1): 39–65, 2006.

166. Lindecrona, R. H., Friis, C. and Nielsen, J. P. Pharmacokinetics and penetration of danofloxacin into the gastrointestinal tract in healthy and in *Salmonella typhimurium* infected pigs. *Research in Veterinary Science*, 68: 211–216, 2000.

167. Liu, P., Fuhrherr, R., Webb, A. I., Obermann, B. and Derendorf, H. Tissue penetration of cefpodoxime into the skeletal muscle and lung in rats. *European Journal of Pharmaceutical Sciences*, 25: 439–444, 2005.

168. Lium, B., Skomsoy, A., Jorgensen, A., Loe, B. and Szancer, J. An attempt to eradicate *Mycoplasma hyopneumoniae* from selected Norwegian farrowing to finishing herds. *Proceedings 12th International Pig Veterinary Society Congress*, The Hague, Holland, p. 300, 1992.

169. Lizarazo, Y. A., Ferri, E. F., De la Fuente, A. J. and Martín, C. B. Evaluation of changes in antimicrobial susceptibility patterns of *Pasteurella multocida* subsp *multocida* isolates from pigs in Spain in 1987-1988 and 2003-2004. *American Journal of Veterinary Research*, 67 (4): 663–8, 2006.

170. Lobova, D., Smola, J. and Cizek, A. Decreased susceptibility to tiamulin and valnemulin among Czech isolates of *Brachyspira hyodysenteriae*. *Journal of Medical Microbiology*, 53, 287–291, 2004.

171. Lode, H., Borner, K. and Koeppe, P. Pharmacodynamics of fluoroquinolones. *Clinical infectious diseases*, 27: 33–39, 1998.

172. Lomax, L. G. and Cole, J. R. Porcine epidermitis and dermatitis associated with *Staphylococcus hyicus* and *Dermatophilus congolensis* infections. *Journal of the American Veterinary Medical Association*, 183: 1091–1092, 1983.

173. Looft, T., Johnson, T. A., Allen, H. K., Bayles, D. O., Alt, D. P., Stedtfeld, R. D., Sul, W. J., Stedtfeld T. M., Chai B., Cole J. R., Hashsham S. A., Tiedje J. M. and Stanton T. B. In-feed antibiotic effects on the swine intestinal microbiome. *Proceedings of the National Academy of Science of the USA*, 109 (5): 1691–6, 2012.

174. López, D., Vlamakis, H. and Kolter, R. Biofilms. *Cold Spring Harb. Perspect. Biol.*, Jul; 2 (7): a000398. doi: 10.1101/cshperspect.a000398. Epub 2010 Jun 2. Review, 2010.

175. Luque, I., Tarradas, C., Carrasco, L., Torroella, E., Artigas, C. and Perea, A. Effectiveness of doxycycline in the prevention of an experimental infection with *Actinobacillus pleuropneumoniae* in pigs. *Journal of Veterinary Medicine B*, 47: 445–451, 2000.

176. MacGowan, A. P. On behalf of the BSAC Working Parties on Resistance Surveillance Clinical implications of antimicrobial resistance for therapy. *Journal of Antimicrobial Chemotherapy*, 62 (suppl 2): ii105–ii114, 2008.

177. MacKinnon, J. D. The proper use and benefits of veterinary antimicrobial agents in swine practice. *Veterinary Microbiology*, 35: 357–367, 1993.

178. MacKenzie, F. M., Bruce, J., Struelens, M. J., Goossens, H., Mollison, J. and Gould I. MARPAC Steering Group. Antimicrobial drug use and infection control practices associated with the prevalence of methicillin-resistant *Staphylococcus aureus* in

European hospitals. *Clinical Microbiology and Infection*, 13: 269–276, 2007.

179. Mackinnon, P. S. and Davis, S. L. Pharmacokinetic and pharmacodynamic issues in the treatment of bacterial infectious diseases. *European Journal of Clinical Microbiology and Infectious Disease*, 23: 271–288, 2004.

180. Maglio, D., Capitano, B., Banevicius, M.A., Geng, Q., Nightingale, C.H. and Nicolau, D. P. Differential efficacy of clarithromycin in lung versus thigh infection models. *Chemotherapy*, 50: 63–66, 2004.

181. Marchant, J. N., Rudd, A. R., Mendl, M. T., Broom, D. M., Meredith, M. J., Corning, S and Simms, P. H. Timing and causes of piglet mortality in alternative and conventional farrowing systems. *Veterinary Record*, 147 pp. 209–214, 2000.

182. Martens, M. G., Maccato, M., Van Hook, C. and Vincent, J. Penetration of trovafloxacin into gynecologic tissues. *American Journal of Surgery*, 176 (6A Suppl): 18S–22S, 1998.

183. Martin, C. E., Hooper, B. E. and Armstrong, C. H. A clinical and pathological study of the mastitis-metritis-agalactia syndrome of sows. *Journal of the American Veterinary Medical Association*, 151: 1629–1634, 1967.

184. Martín-Jiménez, T. and Riviere, J. E. Population pharmacokinetics in veterinary medicine: Potencial use for therapeutic drug monitoring and prediction of tissue residues. *Journal of Veterinary Pharmacology and Therapeutics*, 21: 167–189, 1997.

185. Martín-Jiménez, T. Farmacocinética I: absorción y distribución. In: *Farmacología y terapéutica veterinaria*, Botana L. M., Landoni F., Martín-Jiménez, T. (eds). McGraw-Hill interamericana, 2002.

186. Martín-Jiménez T., McDermott, P. and Walker, R. Pharmacology of the fluorquinolones: A perspective for the use in domestic animals. A review. *Veterinary Journal*, 172 (1): 10–28, 2006.

187. Mateusen, B., Maes, D. Van Goubergen, M., Verdonck, M. and De Kruif, A. Effectiveness of treatment with lincomycin hydrochloride and/or vaccination against *Mycoplasma hypneumoniae* for controlling chronic respiratory disease in a herd of pigs. *Veterinary Record*, 151 (5): 135–140, 2002.

188. Matter, D., Rossano, A., Limat, S., Vorlet-Fawer, L., Brodard, I. and Perreten, V. Antimicrobial resistance profile of *Actinobacillus pleuropneumoniae* and *Actinobacillus porcitonsillarum*. *Veterinary Microbiology*, 122 (1–2): 146–56, 2007.

189. Mauch C. and Bilkei G. The influence of prepartal bacteriuria on the reproductive performance of the sow. *Dtsch Tierarztl Wochenschr*, 111 (4): 166–169, 2004.

190. May, E. R. Bacterial skin diseases: Current thoughts on pathogenesis and management. *Veterinary Clinics of North America: Small Animal Practice*, 36 (1): 185–202, 2006.

191. McKellar, Q. A., Baxter, P., Taylor, D., and Bogan, J. A. Penicillin therapy of spontaneous streptococcal meningitis in pigs. *Veterinary Record*, 121 (15): 347–50, 1987.

192. McKellar, Q. A., Gibson, I., Montero, A. and Bregante, M. Pharmacokinetics of enrofloxacin and danofloxacin in plasma, inflammatory exudate and bronchial secretions of calves following subcutaneous administration. *Antimicrobial Agents and Chemotherapy*, 1988–1992, 1999.

193. McKellar, Q. A., Sanchez Bruni, S. F. and Jones, D. G. Pharmacokinetic/pharmacodynamic relationship of antimicrobial drugs used in veterinary medicine. *Journal of Veterinary Pharmacology and Therapeutics*, 27: 503–514, 2004.

194. McOrist, S., Mackie, R. A. and Lawson, G. H. Antimicrobial susceptibility of ileal symbiont intracellularis isolated from pigs with proliferative enteropathy. *Journal of Clinical Microbiology*, 33 (5): 1314–7, 1995.

195. McOrist, S. Defining the full costs of endemic porcine proliferative enteropathy. *Veterinary Journal*, 170: 8–9, 2005.

196. Merck & Co. *Merck Veterinary Manual*, INC, 1991.

197. Meunier, D., Acar, J. F., Martel, J. L., Kroemer, S. and Valle, M. A seven-year survey of susceptibility to marbofloxacin of pathogenic strains isolated from pets. *International Journal of Antimicrobial agents*, 24: 592–598, 2004.

198. Middleton-Williams D. M., Pohlenz J., Lott-Stolz G. and Bertschinger H. U. Studies on the mastitis-metritis-agalactia syndrome (milk fever) in sows. I. Pathological findings in spontaneous cases. *Schweiz Arch Tierheilkd*, 119 (6): 213–22, 1977.

199. Miller, D. J. S. and Stipkovits, L. Recent advances in the control of enzootic pneumonia in pigs. *Proceedings of the World Veterinary Congress*, Rio de Janeiro, Brazil, 1991.

200. Milligan, B. N., Dewey C. E. and De Grau, A. F. Neonatal-piglet weight variation and its relation to pre-weaning mortality and weight gain on commercial farms. *Preventive Veterinary Medicine*, 56: 119–127, 2002.

201. Molnar, L. Sensitivity of strains of *Serpulina hyodysenteriae* isolated in Hungary to chemotherapeutic drugs. *Veterinary Record*, 138: 158–160, 1996.

202. Moore, R. D., Lietman, P. S. and Smith, C. R. Clinical response to aminoglycoside therapy: importance of the ratio to peak concentration to minimal inhibitory concentration. *Journal of Infectious Diseases*, 155: 93–99, 1987.

203. Morgan, J. H., Aitken, I. A., Collins, P. and Burch, D. G. S. Prevention of experimentally-induced enzootic pneumonia in pigs using the novel compound SDZ PMD 296 (Econor-Sandoz Ltd). *Proceedings 14th International Pig Veterinary Society Congress*, Bologna, Italy, p. 433, 1996.

204. Morkoc, A., Backstrom, L., Lund, L. and Smith, A. R. Bacterial endotoxin in blood of dysgalactic sows in relation to microbial status of uterus, milk, and intestine. *Journal of the American Veterinary Medical Association,* 183: 786–789, 1983.

205. Mouton, J. W. Breakpoints: Current practice and future perspectives. *International Journal of Antimicrobial Agents*, 19: 323–31, 2002.

206. Mouton, J. W. and Vinks, A. A. Pharmacokinetic/pharmacodynamic modelling of antibacterials in vitro and in vivo using bacterial growth and kill kinetics. The minimum inhibitory concentration versus stationary concentration. *Clinical pharmacokinetics*, 44 (2): 201–210, 2005.

207. Mouton, J. W., Ambrose, P. G., Cantón, R., Drusano, G. L., Harbarth, S., Macgowan, A., Theuretzbacher, U. and Turnidge, J. Conserving antibiotics for the future: New ways to use old and new drugs from a pharmacokinetic and pharmacodynamic perspective. *Drug Resistance Update*, 14: 107–11, 2011.

208. Murdoch, M. B. and Peterson, L.R. Antimicrobial penetration into polymorfonuclear leukocytes and alveolar macrophages. *Seminars in Respiratory Infection*, 6 (2): 112–121, 1991.

209. Nachreiner, R. F. and Ginther, O. J. Induction of agalactia by administration of endotoxin (*Escherichia coli*) in swine. *American Journal of Veterinary Research*, 35: 619–622, 1974.

210. National Committee on Clinical Laboratory Standards. *Performance standards for antimicrobial disk and dilution susceptibility test for bacteria isolated from animals. Approved Standard.* NCCLS document M31-A. Wayne, PA: NCCLS, 1999[a].

211. National Committee on Clinical Laboratory Standards. *Development of in vitro susceptibility testing criteria and quality control parameters for veterinary antimicrobial agents. Approved Standard.* NCCLS document M37-A. Wayne, PA: NCCLS, 1999[b].

212. Nathues, H., Holthaus, K. and Beilage, E.G. Quantification of *Lawsonia intracellularis* in porcine faeces by real-time PCR. *Journal of*

Applied Microbiology, 107 (6): 2009–2016, 2009.

213. Nau, R., Kinzig, M, Dreyhaupt, T., Kolenda, H., Sörgel, F. and Prange, H. W. Kinetics of ofloxacin and its metabolites in cerebrospinal fluid after a single intravenous infusion of 400 milligrams of ofloxacin. *Antimicrobial Agents and Chemotherapy*, 38 (8): 1849–53, 1994.

214. Neil, M., Ogle, B. and Annér, K. A two-diet system and ad libitum lactation feeding of the sow 1. Sow performance. *Animal Science*, 62: 337–347, 1996.

215. Nielsen, P. The influence of feed on the oral bioavailability of antibiotics-chemotherapeutics in pigs. *Pharmacology and Therapeutics*, 20 (Suppl. 1): 30–31, 1997.

216. Nishifuji, K., Sugai, M. and Amagai, M. Staphylococcal exfoliative toxins: "molecular scissors" of bacteria that attack the cutaneous defense barrier in mammals. *Journal of Dermatological Science*, 49: 21–31, 2008.

217. Olendorf, W. H. Lipid solubility and drug penetration of the blood-brain barrier. *Proceedings Society Experimental Biology Medicine*, 147: 813–815, 1974.

218. Oliver, S. P., Lewis, T. M., Lewis, H. H., Dowlen, J. L. and Maki, J. L. Persistence of antibiotics in bovine mammary secretions following intramammary infusion at cessation of milking. *Preventive Veterinary Medicine*, 9: 301–311, 1990.

219. Olivry, T. and Linder, K. E. Dermatoses affecting desmosomes in animals: A mechanistic review of acantholytic blistering skin diseases. *Veterinary Dermatology*, 20: 313–326, 2009.

220. Ostergaad, C. *PK/PD properties in bacterial meningitis*. Personal communication, 2005.

221. Owens, W. E., Watts, J. L., Boddie, R. L., and Nickerson, S. C. Antibiotic treatment of mastitis: Comparison of intramamary and intramamary plus intramuscular therapies. *Journal of Dairy Science*, 71: 3143–3147, 1988.

222. Pardridge, W. M. Recent advances in blood-barrier transport. *Annual Review Pharmacology Toxicology*, 28: 25–39, 1988.

223. Pedersen, K. S., Ståhl, M., Guedes, R. M., Angen, O., Nielsen, J. P. and Jensen, T. K. Association between faecal load of *Lawsonia intracellularis* and pathological findings of proliferative enteropathy in pigs with diarrhoea. *BMC Veterinary Research*, 8 (1): 198a, 2012, doi: 10.1186/1746-6148-8-198.

224. Pedersen, K. S., Skrubel, R., Stege, H., Angen, O., Ståhl, M., Hjulsager, C., Larsen, L. E. and Nielsen, J. P. Association between average daily gain, faecal dry matter content and concentration of *Lawsonia intracellularis* in faeces. *Acta Veterinaria Scandinavica*, 54 (1): 58, 2012, doi: 10.1186/1751-0147-54-58.

225. Pejsak, Z. and Tarasuik, K. The occurrence of endotoxin in sows with coliform mastitis. *Theriogenelogy*, 32: 335–341, 1989.

226. Persson, A., Pedersen Morner, A. and Kuhl, W. A long-term study on the health status and performance of sows on different feed allowances during late pregnancy. II. The total cell content and its percentage of polymorphonuclear leucocytes in pathogen-free colostrum and milk collected from clinically healthy sows. *Acta Veterinaria Scandinavica*, 37: 279–291, 1996.

227. Phillips, I., Casewell, M., Cox, T., De Groot, B., Friis C., Jones R., Nightingale C., Preston R. and Waddell, J. Does the use of antibiotics in food animals pose a risk to human health? A critical review of published data. *Journal of Antimicrobial Chemotherapy*, 53: 28–52, 2004.

228. Plumb, D. C. *Veterinary Drug Handbook*, 2nd ed., Iowa State University Press, Ames, USA, 1995.

229. Plumb, D. C. *Veterinary Drug Handbook*, 3rd ed., Iowa State University Press, Ames, USA, 2002.

230. Pluske, J. R., Siba, P. M., Pethick, D. W., Durmic, Z., Mullan, B. P. and Hampson, D. J. The incidence of swine dysentery in pigs can be reduced by feeding diets that limit the amount of fermentable substrate entering

the large intestine. *Journal of Nutrition*, 126 (11): 2920–2933, 1996.

231. Prats, C., El Korchi, G., Giralt, M., Cristofol, C., Peña, J., Zorrilla, I., Saborit, J. and Pérez, B. PK and PK/PD of doxycicline in drinking water after therapeutic use in pigs. *Journal of Veterinary Pharmacology and Therapeutics*, 28: 525–530, 2005.

232. Prescott, J. F. The pathways of resistance transmission. *Antimicrobial Therapy in Veterinary Medicine*. J.F. Prescott et al. (eds), pp. 39. John Wiley & Sons, 1988.

233. Prescott, J. F., Baggot, J. D. and Walker, R. D. *Antimicrobial therapy in veterinary medicine*, 3th ed. Iowa State University Press, Ames, Iowa, 2000.

234. Pringle, M., Landén, A., Unnerstad, H.E., Molander, B. and Bengtsson, B. Antimicrobial susceptibility of porcine *Brachyspira hyodysenteriae* and *Brachyspira pilosicoli* isolated in Sweden between 1990 and 2010. *Acta Veterinaria Scandinavica*, 54 (1): 54, 2012, doi: 10.1186/1751-0147-54-54.

235. Radostits, O. M. Fluoroquinolone resistance trends and animal drug use: a retrospective analysis. *International Journal Infectious Disease*, 8: 187–189, 2004.

236. Rahal, J. J., Urban, C. and Segal-Maurer, S. Nosocomial antibiotic resistance in multiple gram-negative species: experience at one hospital with squeezing the resistance balloon at multiple sites. *Clinical Infectious Disease*, 34: 499–503, 2002.

237. Rasmussen, F. Mammary excretion of benzyl penicillin, erythromycin and penethamate hydriodide. *Acta Pharmacologica et Toxicologica*, 16: 194–200, 1959.

238. Ravel, A., D'Allaire, S. and Bigras-Poulin, M. Influence of management, housing and personality of the stockperson on preweaning performances on independent and integrated swine farms in Quebec. *Preventive Veterinary Medicine*, 29: 37–57, 1996.

239. Rennard, S. I., Basset, G., Lecossier, D., O'Donnell, K. M., Pinkston, P., Martin, P. G. and Crystal, R. G. Estimation of volume of epithelial lining fluid recovered by lavage using urea as marker of dilution. *Journal of Applied Physiology*, 60: 532–538, 1986.

240. *Report of the 3rd meeting of the WHO advisory group on integrated surveillance of antimicrobial resistance*, 14–17 June 2011. Edited by the World Health Organization, 2012.

241. Richter, B., Ladinig, A., Nedorost, N. and Weissenbock, H. A TaqMan quantitative polymerase chain reaction assay for the detection of *Lawsonia intracellularis* in faecal and tissue samples from pigs. *Journal Veterinary Diagnostic Investigation*, 22 (1): 70–73, 2010.

242. Ringarp, N. Clinical and experimental investigation into a postparturient syndrome with agalactia in sows. *Acta Veterinaria Scandinavica*, (Supp 7): 1–153, 1960.

243. Rohde, J., Kessler, M., Baums, C. G., and Amtsberg, G. Comparison of methods for antimicrobial susceptibility testing and MIC values for pleuromutilin drugs for *Brachyspira hyodysenteriae* isolated in Germany. *Veterinary Microbiology*, 102: 25–32, 2004.

244. Ross, R. F., Harmon, R. L., Zimmermann, B.J. and Young, T.F. Susceptibility of sows to experimentally induced *Escherichia coli* mastitis. *American Journal of Veterinary Research*, 44: 949–954, 1983.

245. Rosin, E., Uphoff, T. S., Schultz-Darken, N. J., and Collins, M. T. Cefazolin antibacterial activity and concentrations in serum and the surgical wound in dogs. *American Journal of Veterinary Research*, 54 (8): 1317–1321, 1993.

246. Ross, R. F., Orning, A. P., Woods, R. D., Zimmermann, B. J., Cox, D. F, Harris, D. L. Bacteriologic study of sow agalactia. *American Journal of Veterinary Research*, 42: 949–955, 1981.

247. Rowland, M. and Tozer, T. *Clinical pharmacokinetics. Concepts and applications*. Williams and Wilkins, Media PA, 1995.

248. Sánchez-Rubio, A. and Sánchez Recio, M. M. Basis of anti-infective therapy. Pharmacokinetic-pharmacodynamic criteria and methodology for dual dosage individualisation. *Clinical Pharmacokinetics*, 37 (4): 289–304, 1999.

249. Sarasola, P., Lees, P., Alibaldi, F. S., Mckellar, Q. A., Donachie, W., Marr, K. A., Sunderland, S. J., Rowan, T. G. Pharmacokinetic and pharmacodynamic profiles of danofloxacin administered by two dosing regimens in calves infected with *Mannheimia (Pasteurella haemolytica)*. *Antimicrobial Agents Chemotherapy*, 46 (9): 3013–3019, 2002.

250. Scaglione, F. Can PK/PD be used in everyday clinical practice? *International Journal of antimicrobial agents*, 19: 349–353, 2002.

251. Scaglione, F. and Paraboni, L. Influence of pharmacokinetics/pharmacodynamics of antibacterials in their dosing regimen selection. *Expert Review Antiinfectious Infection Therapy*, 4 (3): 479–490, 2006.

252. Schiønning, S., Millerioux, L., Hewett, G.R. Determination of tissue concentrations of desfuroylceftiofur in pigs after intramuscular injection of Excenel™ sterile powder *Proceedings 6th International Congress of the European Association for Veterinary Pharmacology and Toxicology*, 6 (2): 76. Abstract 012, 1994.

253. Schneider, M., Valle, M., Woehrle, F. and Boisrame, B. Pharmacokinetics of marbofloxacin in lactating cows after repeated intramuscular administrations and pharmacodynamics against mastitis isolated strains. *Journal of Dairy Science*, 87: 202–211, 2004.

254. Schneider, M., Thomas, V., Boisrame, B., and Deleforge, J. Pharmacokinetics of marbofloxacin in dogs after oral and parenteral administration. *Journal Veterinary Pharmacology Therapeutics*, 19: 56–61, 1996.

255. Schuller, von W., Laber, G. and Walzl, H. Chemotherapeutische Untersuchungen mit 81723 hfu (Tiamulin), einem neuen pleuromutilin-derivat, an der experimentellen Mykoplasma-Pneumonie des Schweines. *Deutsche Tierartztliche Wochenschrift*, 9, 345–349, 1977.

256. Scott, D. W., Miller, W. H. and Griffin C.E. *Muller and Kirk's Small Animal Dermatology*, 6th edition. W.B. Saunders, Philadelphia, 2001.

257. Short, C. R. and Clarke, C. R. Calculation of dosage regimens of antimicrobial drugs for the neonatal patient. *Journal of the American Veterinary Medical Association*, 185 (10): 1088–93. 1984.

258. Shryock, T. R. and Richwine, A. The interface between veterinary and human antibiotic use. *Annals of the New York Academic Science*, 1213: 92–105, 2010.

259. Simon, F., Semjen, G., Laczay, P. and Cserep, T. Efficacy of enrofloxacin against enzootic pneumonia in swine. *Proceedings 11th International Pig Veterinary Society Congress*, Lausanne, Switzerland, p. 96, 1990.

260. Smith, S. H. and McOrist, S. Development of persistent intestinal infection and excretion of *Lawsonia intracellularis* by piglets. *Research in Veterinary Science*, 62 (1): 6–10, 1997.

261. Snoeck, V., Huyghebaert, N., Cox, E., Vermeire, A., Saunders, J., Remon, J. P., Vershooten, F. and Goddeeris, B. M. Gastrointestinal transit time of non-disintegrating radio-opaque pellets in suckling and recently weaned piglets. *Journal of Controlled Release*, 94: 143–153, 2004.

262. Ståhl, M., Kokotovic, B., Hjulsager, C. K., Breum, S. Ø. and Angen, Ø. The use of quantitative PCR for identification and quantification of *Brachyspira pilosicoli*, *Lawsonia intracellularis* and *Escherichia coli* fimbrial types F4 and F18 in pig faeces. *Veterinary Microbiology*, 151 (3–4): 307–314, 2011.

263. Sttats, J. J., Feder, I., Okwumabua, O., and Chengappa, M. M. *Streptococcus suis*: Past and present. *Veterinary Research Communications*, 21: 381–407, 1997.

264. Stipkovits, L., Miller, D., Glavits, R., Fodor, L. and Burch, D. Treatment of pigs experimentally infected with *Mycoplasma hyopneumoniae, Pasteurella multocida,* and *Actinobacillus pleuropneumoniae* with various antibiotics. *Canadian Journal of Veterinary Research*, 65: 213–222, 2001.

265. Song, J. H. The goals of antimicrobial therapy. *International Journal of Infectious Disease*, 7: S1–S4, 2003.

266. Straw, B. E., Dewey, C. E. and Wilson, M. R. Differential diagnosis of swine diseases. In: Straw, B. E., D'Allaire, S., Mengeling, W. L. and Taylor, D. J. (eds). *Diseases of Swine*, 8th ed. Ames, Iowa: Iowa State University Press, 521–534, 1999.

267. Sundqvist, M., Geli, P., Andersson, D. I., Sjölund-Karlsson, M., Runehagen, A., Cars, H., Abelson-Storby, K., Cars, O. and Kahlmeter G. Little evidence for reversibility of trimethoprim resistance after a drastic reduction in trimethoprim use. *Journal of Antimicrobial Chemotherapy*, 65: 350–360, 2010.

268. Suzuki, H., Terasaki, T., Sugiyama, Y. Role of efflux transport across the blood-brain barrier and blood-cerebroespinal fluid barrier on the disposition of xenobiotics in the central nervous system. *Advanced Drug Delivery Review*, 25: 257–285, 1997.

269. Szancer, J. Eradication programmes for swine dysentery. *International Pig Topics*, 20 (8): 7–9, 2005.

270. Takasugi, N., Tsunaga, N., Sugino, N., Numa, F. and Kato, H. Penetration of cefpodoxime into uterine and vaginal secretions from postpartum women after a single oral dose of cefpodoxime proxetil. *Antimicrobial Agents Chemotherapy*, 40 (8): 1832–1834, 1996.

271. Tamma, P. D. and Cosgrove S. E. Antimicrobial stewardship. *Infectious Disease Clinical North America*, 25: 245–260, 2011.

272. Taylor, D. J. *Pig Diseases*, 8th ed. Glasgow: DJ Taylor, 220–223, 2006.

273. Ter Laak, E.A., Pijpers, A., Noordergraaf, J.H., Schoevers, E.C. and Verheijden, J.H.M. Comparison of methods for in vitro testing of susceptibility of porcine mycoplasma species to antimicrobial agents, *Antimicrobial Agents Chemotherapy*, 35: 228–233, 1991.

274. Ter Laak, E. A., Noordergraaf J. H., andVerschure M. H. Susceptibilities of *Mycoplasma bovis, Mycoplasma dispar* and *Ureaplasma diversum* strains to antimicrobial agents in vitro. *Antimicrobial Agents Chemotherapy*, 37, 317–321, 1993.

275. Threlfall, W. R., Martin, C. E. Swine agalactia in Missouri. *Veterinary Medicine and Small Animal Clinician*, 68: 423–426, 1973.

276. Thacker, E., Thacker, B. and Wolff, T. Efficacy of Aureomycin chlortetracycline against experimental *Mycoplasma hyopneumoniae* challenge. *Proceedings 16th International Pig Veterinary Society Congress*, Melbourne, Australia, p. 457, 2000.

277. Theuretzbacher, U. Protein binding and tissue concentrations. Do they matter? *8th ISAP Educational Workshop*, Glasgow, 2003.

278. Tzipori, D., Chandler, D., Smith, M., Makin, T. and Hennessy, D. Factors contributing to postweaning diarrhoea in a large intensive piggery. *Australian Veterinary Journal*, 56: 74–278, 1980.

279. Toutain, P. L., Del Castillo, J. R. E. and Bousquet-Melou, A. The pharmacokinetic-pharmacodynamic approach to a rational dosage regimen for antibiotics. *Research in Veterinary Science*, 73: 105–114, 2002.

280. Toutain, P. L. and Bousquet-Melou, A. Plasma clearance. *Journal of Veterinary Pharmacology and Therapeutics*, 27: 414–425, 2004a.

281. Toutain, P. L. and Bousquet-Melou, A. Volumes of distribution. *Journal of Veterinary*

Pharmacology and Therapeutics, 27: 441–453, 2004[b].

282. Toutain, P. L. and Bousquet-Melou, A. Plasma terminal half-life. *Journal of Veterinary Pharmacology and Therapeutics*, 27: 427–439, 2004[c].

283. Toutain, P. L. and Bousquet-Melou, A. Bioavailability and its assesment. *Journal of Veterinary Pharmacology and Therapeutics*, 27: 455–466, 2004[d].

284. Toutain, P. L and Lees, P. Integration and modelling of pharmacokinetic and pharmacodynamic data to optimize dosage regimens in veterinary medicine. *Journal of Veterinary Pharmacology and Therapeutics*, 27: 467–477, 2004[e].

285. Turnidge, J., Paterson, D. L. Setting and revising antibacterial susceptibility breakpoints. *Clinical Microbiology Reviews*, 20: 391–408, 2007.

286. Valderrey, A. D., Pozuelo, M. J., Jiménez, P. A., Maciá, M. D., Oliver, A. and Rotger, R. Chronic colonization by *Pseudomonas aeruginosa* of patients with obstructive lung diseases: cystic fibrosis, bronchiectasis, and chronic obstructive pulmonary disease. *Diagnostic Microbiology and Infectious Disease*, 68 (1): 20–27, 2010.

287. Van Beers-Schreurs, H. M. G, Vellenga, L., Wensing, T. and Breukink, H. J. The pathogenesis of the post-weaning syndrome in weaned piglets; a review. *Veterinary Quarterly*, 14: 29–34, 1992.

288. Van Bree, J. B., De Boer, A. G., Danhof, M., Ginsel, L. A. and Breimer, D. D. Characterization of an "in vivo" blood-brain barrier: Effects of molecular size and lipophilicity on cerebrovascular endothelial transport rates of drugs. *Journal of Veterinary Pharmacology and Therapeutics*, 247: 1233–1239, 1988.

289. Van Duijkeren, E., Jansen, M. D. and Flemming, S. C. Methicillinresistant *Staphylococcus aureus* in pigs with exudative epidermitis. *Emerging Infectious Disease*, 13: 1408–1410, 2007.

290. Vicca, J., Stankenborg, T., Maes, D., Butaye, P., Peeters, J., Kruif, A. D. and Haesebrouck, F. In vitro susceptibilities of *Mycoplasma hyopneumoniae* field isolates. *Antimicrobial Agents and Chemotherapy*, 48 (11): 4470–4472, 2004.

291. Villarino N., Lesman, S., Fielder, A., García-Tapia, D., Cox, S., Lucas, M., Robinson J., Brown, S.A. and Martín-Jiménez, T. Pulmonary pharmacokinetics of tulathromycin in swine. Part I: Lung homogenate in healthy pigs and pigs challenged intratracheally with lipopolysaccharide of *Escherichia coli*. *Journal of Veterinary Pharmacology and Therapeutics*, doi: 10.1111/jvp.12016. [Epub ahead of print], 2012.

292. Villarino, N., Lesman, S., Fielder, A., García-Tapia D., Cox, S., Lucas M., Robinson, J., Brown, S. A. and Martín-Jiménez, T. Pulmonary pharmacokinetics of tulathromycin in swine. Part 2: Intra-airways compartments. *Journal of Veterinary Pharmacology and Therapeutics*, doi: 10.1111/jvp.12015. [Epub ahead of print], 2012.

293. Waller, C. M., Bilkei, G. and Cameron, R. D. Effect of periparturient diseases accompanied by excessive vulval discharge and weaning to mating interval on sow reproductive performance. *Austrian Veterinary Journal*, 80 (9): 545–549, 2002.

294. Wallgren, P., Vallgarda, M., Lindberg, L., Eliasson-Selling, L. and Segall, T. Experimental infections with *Actinobacillus pleuropneumoniae* in pigs II: Comparison of antibiotics for oral strategic treatment. *Journal of Veterinary Medicine B*, 46: 261–269, 1999.

295. Walker, R. D. Antimicrobial susceptibility testing and interpretation of results. In Prescott, J. F., Baggot, J. D. and Walker, R.D. *Antimicrobial therapy in veterinary medicine*, 3th ed. Iowa State University Press, Ames, Iowa, 2000.

296. Wattanaphansak, S., Singer, R. S. and Gebhart, C. J. In vitro antimicrobial activity against 10 North American and European

Lawsonia intracellularis isolates. *Veterinary Microbiology*, 134 (3–4): 305-10, 2009.

297. Wattanaphansak, S., Gebhart, C. J., Anderson, J. M. and Singer, R. S. Development of a polymerase chain reaction assay for quantification of *Lawsonia intracellularis*. *Journal of Veterinary Diagnostic Investigation*, 22 (4): 598–602, 2010.

298. Wegmann, P., Bertschinger, H. U. and Jecklin, H. A field study on the prevalence of coliform mastitis (MMA syndrome) in Switzerland and the antimicrobial susceptibility of the coliform bacteria from the milk. *8th International Pig Veterinary Society Congress*, Barcelona, Spain, p. 92, 1986.

299. Wegener, H. C., Watts, J. L., Salmon, S. A. and Yancey, R. J. Antimicrobial susceptibility of *Staphylococcus hyicus* isolated from exudative epidermitis in pigs. *Journal Clinical Microbiology*, 132 (3): 793–795, 1994.

300. Wegener, H. C. and Skov-Jensen, E. W. Exudative epidermitis. In: Straw B. E., Zimmerman J. J., D'Allaire S et al. (eds). *Diseases of Swine*, 9th ed. Ames, IA: Blackwell Publishing. 675–679, 2006.

301. Whittem, T. and Gaon, D. Principles of antimicrobial therapy. *Veterinary Clinics North American Small Animal Practice*, 28 (2): 197–213, 1998.

302. Winkelman, N., Evans, R.A. and Cornell, C.P. *Proceedings of the 15th International Pig Veterinary Society Congress*, Birmingham, England, p. 195, 1998.

303. Winkelman, N. *Proceedings 30th American Association of Swine Practitioners Meeting*, St. Louis, Missouri, USA, p. 241–242, 1999.

304. Wisselink, H.J., Smith H.E., Stockhofe-Zurwieden, N., Peperkamp, K. and Vecht, U. Distribution of capsular types and production of muramidase-released protein (MRP) and extracellular factor (EF) of *Streptococcus suis* strains isolated from diseased pigs in seven European countries. *Veterinary Microbiology*, 74 (3), 237–248, 2000.

305. Wisselink, H.J., Veldman, K.T., Van den Eede, C., Salmon, S.A., Mevius, D.J.. Quantitative susceptibility of *Streptococcus suis* strains isolated from diseased pigs in seven European countries to antimicrobial agents licensed in veterinary medicine. *Veterinary Microbiology*, 113 (1–2): 73–82, 2006.

306. Yancey, R. J., Evans, R. A., Kratzer, D. D., Paulissen, J. B. and Carmer, S. G. Efficacy of ceftiofur hydrochloride for treatment of experimentally induced colibacilosis in neonatal swine. *American Journal Veterinary Research*, 51 (3): 349-353, 1990.

307. Zhao, X. and Drlica, K. A unified antimutant dosing strategy. *Journal of Antimicrobial Chemotherapy*, 62: 434–436, 2008.

308. Yamaoka, K. Statistical moments in pharmacokinetics. *Journal of Pharmacokinetic Biopharmacy*, 6 (6): 547, 1978.

309. Ziv, G. Drug selection and use in mastitis: systemic versus local drug therapy. *Journal of the American Veterinary Medical Association*, 176: 1109–115, 1980[a].

310. Ziv, G. Practical pharmacokinetic aspects of mastitis therapy-2- Practical and therapeutic applications. *Agri Practice*, 469–476, 1980 [b].

311. Ziv, G. Practical pharmacokinetic aspects of mastitis therapy-3- Intrammary treatment. *Veterinary Medicine/Small Animal Clinic*. April 1980 [c].

312. Ziv, G, Storper, M. Intramuscular treatment of subclinical staphylococcal mastitis in lactating cows with penicillin G, methillin and their esters. *Journal of Veterinary Pharmacology and Therapeutics*, 8: 276–283, 1985.

Published by Servet editorial - Grupo Asís Biomedia S.L.